The Adventur

Cont

I dedicate this book to my brother Micheal

Christopher Button

The events in this book document my time as a newly qualified nurse from 2015-2016. All the names of the patients I cared for, and the staff I worked with, have been anonymized to maintain confidentiality

CHAPTER 1: TRANSITION TO NEWLY QUALIFIED NURSE

My journey to becoming a registered nurse was one of the most difficult challenges of my life. I started my training at the age of twenty-four, and I felt like I was still emerging as an adult, trying to find my way in life.

Throughout my journey as a student nurse, I worked in many different areas, including a cardiac ward, a district community nursing service, an accident and emergency department and a stroke ward. I found so many areas of nurse training difficult, such as learning to communicate with difficult patients, coping with difficult mentors who despised student nurses, and trying to juggle full-time work, whilst also completing the academic requirements of my course.

Throughout my nurse training, I was carrying a deep heartache inside of me. At the start of my training, my identical twin brother Michael was diagnosed with an inoperable brain tumor. In between completing twelve-hour shifts and writing assignments, I helped to care for my brother and helped to improve the quality of his life. By the end of my training, Michael had passed away.

After Michael's death, I discovered a range of letters he had written and 'wishes' he had created for me in the event of his death. Michael had requested for me to follow my childhood dream and to become an actor.

Following Michael's wishes, I made the decision to travel to New York to audition for the role of the scarecrow in 'The Wizard of Oz' production. In the role of the scarecrow, I traveled around different areas of America, such as Florida, Los Angeles, and Texas, performing to sell-out crowds, and achieving great reviews. Financially I was making enough money to live comfortably, and I made a great group of friends, but I missed my parents and life at home.

I had always enjoyed the caring nature of being a nurse and making a difference in people's lives. My life as a trainee nurse was filled with so many challenges, I felt like I was juggling in order to complete all the tasks required in a 12-hour shift. At one point I would be administering medications, at another time I could be caring for a patient suffering from a terminal illness, to saving someone's life through completing CPR.

Each day in the ward, and in the community, was different from the next day, and it was a challenge I wanted to take on, to transition from a student nurse to a nurse.

Working as a student nurse had set the foundation for my future. I had experienced so many new situations. I held the hand of a dying woman, I saved a young man's life as he went into cardiac arrest, I ducked and dived from a lady who was intending on throwing sharp utensils at me. The hardest part of my nurse training was saying goodbye to my twin brother Michael.

I started my nurse training as nervous twenty-four-year-old, naive and unaware of the outside world. I finished my training as a different person, assertive, confident and self-aware of others around me, my life changed forever.

CHAPTER 2: MY FIRST DAY

I arrived back at my family home in Yorkshire after an eleven-hour plane journey. As I arrived home the house looked so different, so empty, and lonely without my brother Michael. Memories of my brother filled the entire house. A Picture of us surfing on the beach in Northumberland on our eighteenth birthday hung above the grand fireplace, whilst our graduation photos were placed on the mantelpiece.

My parents had traveled to New York for a year, and left the house for me to look after. I had just gained a rotational post as a band five nurse post at a local Yorkshire hospital. The post included rotating around different areas including a stroke ward, a cardiac ward, an accident and emergency department, and a nursing telephone advisor phone line.

My brand new uniform had arrived and it hung in the wardrobe ready for the morning. The dark blue uniform was a symbol of how far I have come, whilst the bright white uniform I wore as a student symbolized that I was inexperienced and lacked expertise. I never agreed with wearing different colored uniforms, I felt that all nurses regardless of training and level of experience should wear the same uniform. Uniforms can be seen as having a negative connotation and segregated staff, and this was further influenced by staff who would change their whole personality once they gained promotion and had to wear a different color uniform.

I woke up at 6 am and sat apprehensively eating my lumpy porridge, sitting in my blue uniform, thinking of all the tasks I would need to undertake, and hoping I would fit into my new environment. I packed my satchel with a litre of cold water, five cheese sandwiches, and chocolate biscuits.

I then made the apprehensive walk to Yorkshire hospital, down the long scenic country road. It was bitterly cold, my hands felt frozen, and I began to shiver as I made my way down the steep hill. I wanted to be perfect, I wanted to prove to my preceptor that I was able to complete my competencies and pass. I arrived at the hospital at 6 am, Yorkshire county hospital was a small community hospital where every member of staff knew each other, and a friendly atmosphere greeted you as soon as you entered the building.

I arrived at the staff room in the stroke ward at 7 am. As I walked through the door I heard the same recurring noises, the beeping from the observation machines, the siren from the call buzzer, The shout of patients calling 'nurse!' 'nurse!' and watching as the night staff zoom around the ward, completing their tasks preparing for handover.

As I made my way to the staff room I was greeted by Dana the ward sister. Dana was a warm, kind, and caring person, who made sure she greeted each patient and rushed around to help each nurse and healthcare assistant who required help. "Chris it's so wonderful to have you on our team," she beamed, hugging me tightly. It was then that Dana introduced me to my Preceptor, a nurse who I would work alongside in my first few weeks on the ward. The nurse was called Hayley Ryan. Haley was six foot five with long blonde curly hair, she would constantly leave the ward to smoke a cigarette, and would swear constantly through the shift. I didn't realize at the time but Hayley was happy to support me so that she could offload work on to me.

I was overwhelmed by sitting in the handover room, listening to the tired night nurse handover the five male patients I would be looking after in bay A with complex needs.
The first patient was David a fifty-year-old man, who was over eighteen stone, and suffered a stroke at London Houston station. David was unable to move in the bed and the stroke affected his speech. The doctors explained that David's stroke may have been linked to his unhealthy lifestyle of eating junk food and his lack of exercise. David requires immediate physiotherapy input and occupational therapy assistance.
The second patient was Clive a ninety five-year-old man who previously had a stroke, and was admitted following increased confusion. Clive required one to one supervision from a healthcare assistant, as he kept on trying to walk on his own, but his mobility was very poor and he was at a high risk of falling due to his unsteady gait. On his table, he had a range of activities such as coloring books and puzzles to provide him with cognitive stimu-

lation to improve his well being.

The third patient was Liam a fifty-five-year-old man who doctors believed had a series of TIA strokes due to his alcohol addiction. Liam was admitted to the ward over a month ago. Liam became very angry throughout his stay, constantly expressing that he wanted to go home. Liam had refused to have input with the physiotherapy team, meaning he was unable to mobilize and improve his wellbeing following the stroke.

The fourth patient was a man who had suffered from a trans ischemic stroke and developed respiratory failure following his hospital admission for Pneumonia. Arnold was eighty-nine years old and was receiving palliative care, after the doctors gave him a week to live. Arnold was nursed behind a closed blue curtain. Arnold lay in his electrical bed and had oxygen via nasal specs to give him comfort in his final days. Arnold always had his family around him, sitting around his bed with warm drinks, holding his hand to offer him emotional comfort.

The fifth patient was Sean a forty-two-year-old man who had made a full recovery from his stroke, and was able to mobilize with a walking stick following complete immobility six weeks previously.

After the handover, I walked out nervously towards my bay. In my first shift, I was working with two other nurses Vicki a nurse who completed extra shifts whilst training to become a midwife, and Steven a fifty-five-year-old man, who trained as a nurse in the Philippines and was highly skilled.

I walked nervously into my bay, "Good morning everyone I am Chris I will be looking after you!" I beamed. The patients did not respond. As I looked into the bay the five men were fast asleep and were soon woken up by the healthcare assistants to prepare for their breakfast.

Hayley stormed into the bay with her large medication trolley, "C'mon Chris time to give out the medications!" she groaned. Hayley was the type of nurse who believed in giving medications and completing paperwork, but would never provide personal care to a patient. If she had not been supervising me she would have carelessly left the tablets on the patient's table expecting them to take the tablets themselves. I managed to administer the medications correctly to the patients, making sure I checked the accuracy and correct dosage.

As soon as the medications were completed Hayley disappeared out of the ward for her first cigarette out of one thousand that she would smoke in shifts, constantly leaving the bay.

I began to help Christie the forty-year-old healthcare assistant to complete the daily washes. Our first Patient was David a 55-year-old patient who was over eighteen stone. A week before he had traveled to America for a meeting as part of his director position for Apple. When he arrived at California airport he suffered a major stroke.

David struggled to turn in the bed, and as he turned towards me, Christine had to help with all her strength lifting up his limbs to make sure he was thoroughly cleaned. As we began to wash David, tears rolled down his cheek. "I feel so useless I feel like cabbage, I'll never be able to work again, he cried."

"You have to keep positive, It will take time to recover but if you work with physiotherapists and occupational therapists we can get you moving again," I smiled. We slowly helped David get changed into his day clothes, before using a hoist to help him into the chair. We hoisted David into the chair and supported his weaker right side with pillows. It can be very difficult for patients who suffer from a stroke to remain positive as depression is a common side effect. David was very depressed, So I always remained positive to him, giving him gentle prompts and words of encouragement to help him to engage with therapists to overcome his reluctance.

It was then that I and Christine helped Arnold to have a wash. Arnold was at the end stage of his condition and required full assistance with his wash. The family had filled the room with pictures that detailed memories of his life. A picture of him in his army clothes standing next to his wife on his wedding day was in a silver frame by the window. Whilst another, photo by his bedside was a picture of him in the cockpit in his role as a pilot, his career of forty years. It was an honor to look after patients in the final stage of their life, it was very rewarding to work with my team to help provide as much comfort to Arnold as he needed. In his room, Arnold listened to classic songs by singers such as Buddy Holly and Elvis, which brought back great memories to him of the dances he would attend with his wife in his post-war days.

We then proceeded to wash Clive who was suffering from Dementia. "Who the fuck are you two?" he shouted. "Hi, Clive it's me and Christine We are part of the nursing staff looking after you," I smiled. "You look more like Laurel and Hardy to me!" he scowled. Clive had a range of activities to help support him with his dementia condition such as a coloring book, a special feely bag filled with a bouncy ball, a Cubic cube and a pack of cards, to help support the cognitive stimulation he needed. We proceeded to help Clive offering encouragement, and he was able to follow prompts. "Oh, Clive you're doing so well, with your wash!" I smiled. "You patronizing bastard!" he scowled, before grabbing the large bowl of water and throwing it all over Christine, whilst I successfully ducked. We helped Clive to sit in the chair, although his walking was unsteady, his behavior became very erratic, so we had to arrange for an agency carer to provide one to one support to him. As soon as Clive sat in the chair, he attempted to get up and walk to his car, however, Clive was unable to walk safely on his own, and required constant assistance and supervision from the agency nurse.

It was always so hard to see patients with dementia on a stroke ward, it was nor a conducive environment, and instead made patients feel further confused.

I then walked over to Liam's bedside and he lay angrily in the bed holding onto his arms, he was suffering from deep depression. As we assisted Liam with the wash, he began to hit out angrily at us, "I don't want to be here! I want to go home!" he shouted, attempting to punch Christie "Liam we need to help you, please don't hit us," I requested. It was then that he started to cry hysterically, he fell so trapped, so angry, and hitting out at us was a way of venting his anger. It was then that Liam nodded and consented to us helping him into his wheelchair. We used the hoist to help Liam into the wheelchair. As soon as he sat in his wheelchair, Liam's two daughters Elaine and Rachel entered the bay, to take their Dad outside, he was so angry.

It was then that I completed the doctor's ward round, with the consultant Mrs. Shake who would dress in eccentric outfits such as a leather suit, a lavish dress, or a biker jacket with platform shoes. Today she wore a black dress with resembled a big bag. Mrs. Shake then gave me a list of tasks to be completed, such as discharging Sean and getting his tablets ready. I had to refer Liam to a rehab hospital, arrange a meeting with the palliative care team to discuss home care for Arnold, encourage David to attend physiotherapy sessions, and a care home manager was coming to assess the suitability, of having Clive stay at his specialized care home.

Hayley returned after all the washes had been completed, she smelled of cigarettes and explained that she felt tired, even though she had only completed the medications. I watched Dana as she zoomed around the ward, helping patients to the toilet, and working hard to help complete tasks for the stressed burned-out nurses. Hayley zoomed into the bay reluctantly helping to fill in the paperwork. It was now 12, three hours had passed so fast.

I went into the staffroom for my break leaving the bay of patients in the hands of Hayley and Christine. I sat in the small secluded staffroom, eating my cheese and crackers. Life in the hospital was so different from my life as an actor. As an actor, I was constantly calm and performed with a surge of nervous energy. The wards always felt like a pressure cooker, understaffed, noisy, full of drama, but watching patients recover was so rewarding.

My half an hour break seemed to end so quickly. I walked back onto the ward and witnessed Hayley leaning across the nurse's station as if she was in a bar telling jokes. Christine and the agency nurse Beth decided to take their break so I was on my own.
I looked on in disbelief as I walked into the bay, Clive stood in the middle of the bay unsteadily dressed in his suit carrying his half-open suitcase filled with clothes he had stolen from Arnold's cupboard. "Clive come and walk back with me to your bed space," I

said, attempting to encourage him back to his chair. "No I have to go we are heading out to France tomorrow morning, and I need to meet the other soldiers tomorrow," he insisted. Clive believed he was seventeen and back to his days as a soldier. "Where's my tablet's? I've been waiting for five hours!" Sean shouted. "Sean Your tablets will be ready soon I'm a little ahhhhhhhhh" I screamed. Clive had decided to bite my hand in anger, "Let me out of this prison you bastard, wait till my General finds you, you'll be in for it!" he scowled. I shouted for Hayley to come and help me, and she lazily walked towards me, helping Clive to sit in his armchair. "If my tablets are not here in the next hour I'm going!" Sean shouted.

Suddenly the Physiotherapist assistant called me to the therapy Gym in the ward to witness David's physiotherapy treatment session. As I walked into the gym I looked on in disbelief, David was walking with the physiotherapists for the first time since his stroke occurred over two months ago. "I'm doing it, Chris, I'm walking! I never thought I could!" He beamed. It was so positive to see, after a month of battling to help David participate in his therapy sessions he was finally walking with the assistance of a walking frame. David believed that he would never be able to return to his high profile job, but he finally appeared more positive. It was the best part of working on a stroke ward, watching when patients were regaining their mobility and were beginning to make a recovery.

It was 1 pm and time for visitors to enter the ward for two hours. It was a very overwhelming time, nurses seemed to congregate around the nurses' station, whilst family members approached us with hundreds of questions. Sean's wife questioned me as to why his tablets were taking so long to come up, whilst Liam's family explained that they wanted to make a complaint regarding missing items from his locker, and Clive's wife wanted to ask if she could stay for dinner. Family-centered care is very important in the hospital, but visiting time seemed to make the bays feel like cluttered train stations, filled with people feeling a range of mixed emotions, I reveled in pulling the bell to ask them to leave.

I felt so tired that afternoon, I did not sit down all day, and there were so many tasks to complete, another medication round, notes, referrals, and a social worker meeting. I felt so overwhelmed on my first day, and Hayley seemed to have smoke steam evaporating from her hair, she incessantly left the ward to have a cigarette.

As I walked into the bay, I saw a rare but wonderful sight for a nurse in a busy ward, to see all the patients sitting in their chairs or in their beds settled. Sean sat in his chair, folding his arms, refusing to hold his stare as he became angry waiting for his tablets. Sean sat in his armchair holding the hands of his wife Bridget, "This is my Mum Mr, she's coming to drive me to the dock for our journey to the battle of the Somme," he smiled. "I'm not your mum dear I'm your wife," she smiled.
"Can Clive stay here for a few more weeks he loves it here," Bridget claimed. "It's probably too confusing for Clive to stay here, it would suit him better in his home environment," I insisted.

I then took the rare opportunity to sit with Arnold whilst his family were away, He squeezed onto my hand as I took a seat next to him. "Thank you for all you've done for me and for supporting my family!" he smiled. "If there's anything you want, please tell me," I smiled. "I just want to go home, spend my final few days in my bedroom at home overlooking our farmland." I will speak to the palliative care team and express your request to them," I smiled. Arnold began to squeeze my hand tighter, crying in pain, before I administered Morphine to him to help alleviate his pain. I walked over to Liam as his daughters sat angrily next to him, I could feel their icy cold stares dig into me. "When can Dad come home? He really is sick of being here, we do not seem to be progressing!" Karen cried. It was then that I took a seat next to Liam and his daughters and drew the curtains around his bed space to have a private conversation with the family. "Liam we really feel you need to speak to our hospital rapid mental health team. Over the past month you have refused to mobilize or to work with our therapists, the mental health team, just want to support your wellbeing, I understand that you feel depressed, but I want you to know that there is help there for you." I breathed a sigh of despair as I looked on at a depressed Liam clenched up in the bed, angrily, refusing to look me in the eye. It was one of the hardest parts of being a nurse, watching a patient who really needs help refuse care.

It was then that a stressed Hayley walked over to me, her curly hair standing on end, her uniform stunk of cigarettes, "Chris I'm so sorry I have to go home, I'm feeling really sick," Hayley moaned before exiting the ward. I couldn't believe it my first shift as a student nurse, and the nurse supervising me disappeared.
Once Hayley left the ward I had to gain support from Dana the ward Sister, who was constantly busy and attending to the other nurses' queries simultaneously.

Mealtime arrived on the ward and the bell rang for the visitors to leave the ward. Finally, I could breathe for the first time in the shift. Clive was being supported by his wife, and Christine assisted me in making the patients comfortable and in getting them sitting comfortably for dinner.

I then helped the staff distribute the meals to the patients. The female bays were quiet and peaceful compared to my chaotic bay. The other nurses seemed so calm and relaxed, I tried to display confidence but inside I was terrified of making a mistake.
I distributed the meals carefully to the men in my bay. Sean sat angrily in his chair, refusing his sandwich, he had waited over four hours for his medication and was threatening to leave the ward. Clive was arguing with his wife, complaining that he wanted ice cream instead of the roast dinner. I sat with Liam, as he began to eat the mashed potatoes motionless, with no expression. I tried to prompt him, but he was so depressed and only managed to eat

a few spoonfuls. Christine sat in a chair next to David assisting him with his dinner. I only had two hours left of the shift and I still had many tasks to complete including completing fluid and diet charts, recording patient notes, and then handing over to the night staff. I was still the new person in the ward, with a lot to prove, but knowing I could return to my job as an actor which I enjoyed and thrived in.

Suddenly Clive catapulted his food in the air and then roast potatoes landed on Liam's bed. "You bastard don't throw food at me!" Liam shouted.
"I need to go, I have to be up tomorrow for army training at 6 am, I have to get out of this prison," he roared. Clive's wife Helena attempted to hold his hand to calm him down, but he proceeded to throw his water jug and toiletries on the floor. It was then that Sister Dana intervened, and gently walked over to Clive and held his hand with in an instant his mood changed. Dana's soft voice, calm exterior and forty years of experience showed in the way that she was able to help resolve difficult situations.

"How can I help Clive to feel more relaxed in this environment I hate seeing him swear and bing so aggressive, he is a Christian man," she cried. "Well, you can support him through bringing in familiar objects from home, photos, and games to help him to reminisce which can help elevate his low mood."
I looked over to Paul's space, and he had left a note on his table, 'sick of waiting will come back to the ward to collect tablets tomorrow.' As Dana completed my medications, I hurriedly completed my nursing notes, whilst drinking a cup of hot chocolate. My first drink of the day at 6 pm!

Clive's Wife returned an hour later with a bag full of items. In the bag, she had a collection of his war medals and a photo album that contained photos of key periods in his life. The photos included a picture of him on his wedding day, whilst another photo showed him waving goodbye to his wife on the express train before he left to join the army at seventeen. Other items in the bag included a soft teddy bear and an assortment of sweets. Instantly I noticed a change in Clive's behavior, once he received the items, he appeared more relaxed and calm, the pictures brought back memories for him. Looking at old and familiar items is part of a term called reminiscence therapy, which can help patients who have dementia in making them feel more settled and relaxed.

I felt so tired I was nearing the end of my shift, I constantly heard my name being called by patients and staff, I felt I was drowning in a sea of the list of tasks I had to complete. I helped Christine hoist David and Liam back to bed, and we checked their continence pad to make sure they felt comfortable. Lastly, we helped to reposition Arnold who required strict two-hourly turns to keep his skin clean and to check for any pressure sores.

Arnold's brother Sean arrived and sat with him, holding his hand, as he struggled to keep his eyes open. Watching Arnold's interaction with his brother resembled my own relationship with my brother Michael. When I started my course he was diagnosed with grade four brain cancer. When I returned home from University in the later stages of illness, I would sit with him as he lay on the bed, telling him about my day, and talking about our previous holiday to America. I always felt like I lost my brother too soon, he died suddenly collapsing in a supermarket on his way to visit me. After he died I received various envelopes from Michael in the event of his passing. Inside the enveloped included keys to his Mercedes cars, money, and keys to my Grandparent's cottage which he renovated in Northumberland. On the day of the first shift I thought about Michael less, I almost felt guilty. For over a year each day, I would carry with me a sense of loneliness. I instantly wanted to call him and ask for advice, and it was so hard now that he was gone.

It was then that a new patient arrived called Jack had arrived, with his wife Martha. Jack was admitted with confusion after he spent two hours driving around a roundabout for over two hours, and his wife stated that his behavior has worsened following the death of his mother. As soon as I met Jack he asked me to help him to the toilet. As he stood up he struggled to stand and collapsed instantly on the floor, I then had to use a hoist with Christine to help him onto the commode, and then onto the bed. I then had to complete an incident report which took one hour to complete.

My shift had finally finished and I found it so challenging, adjusting to life as a newly qualified nurse, and having the responsibility of looking after my own patients, even if my preceptor had decided to leave halfway through my shift.

I then had to hand over to the night staff the tasks to be completed on the shift for the patients. I handed over that Arnold needed to have the transport team ready by 10 am the next day, to take him home where he would receive palliative care at home. David required more physiotherapy intervention, and a home visit was required to check the safety of his home. I had arranged for Liam to speak to the hospital mental health team to help alleviate his low mood, whilst I explained that Clive required constant supervision due to his confusion, and had to be visited by two nursing home manager's to assess the suitability of him living there.

CHAPTER 3: THE LIFT

I woke up the next morning at 6 am, and I crept downstairs to make myself some warm golden oats porridge and orange juice. As I sat at the kitchen table I looked outside watching the early morning sun right in a golden haze of orange and yellow light. I wore my wool parka jacket over my nurses' uniform and made my way down the long country road. It was another bitterly cold morning, and I could feel my hands start to go numb as the frost reached the tip of my fingers. My walk to work was a stark contrast to life in New York, gone were the people rushing past me on the sidewalk, the beeping from the yellow taxis, and the shouts and screams from people passing by. As I walked down the beautiful scenic country roads, I could hear the chirping of the birds in the sycamore tree, and the whistling of the branches as I made my way to work. I thought about my brother that morning imagining where he would be if he was twenty-seven. I believed he would have progressed in his position as a doctor and reached the level of consultant eventually, and I know he always wanted to have his own children and to marry one day.

I reached the hospital at 6:40 pm ready and nervous for my shift hoping that the staff on we're going to help me and support me during the shift.

I made my way to the lift and proceeded to enter. "Morning everyone," I smiled, to the other in the lift. The lift was filled with a range of familiar and new faces, including the seventy-year-old porter John with a wispy gray beard and black thick glasses. Then there was a young nurse Gabrielle with a confused elderly lady in a hospital wheelchair heading to X-ray. The other nurse was Katie who was in my cohort of nurses when I trained. Then there was a middle-aged couple Sheila and Thomas who were visiting Clive my previous patient on the stroke ward.

I remember thinking how strange it was that the lift was taking so long to reach the top. Then the lift jolted and the doors wouldn't open and I started to panic. "What's going on? I need the toilet!" shouted the old lady. "Don't worry I've been in this lift before, sometimes the doors get jammed. It only lasts for a few seconds," he smiled. After a few minutes, we all waited silently, "Oh no I really need to be in work today I have my medical examination at 10!" Katie whined.

"C'mon Chris help me open up doors, you hold the top end and I'll prise the bottom of the lift," said John the porter. As I helped John to open the door it worked to no avail as the doors were sealed shut. "Open the door I'm desperate I'm going to wet myself! Here I'll try and open it!" shouted the old lady, as she grabbed her walking stick and began to smash the entrance of the lift, before a worried Gabrielle grabbed the stick, and in a state of panic, pressed the emergency alarm, but it was broken!

We had only been stuck in the lift for ten minutes but that was enough to cause great hysteria and panic for the others in the lift. Suddenly we heard the security team outside, with words of comfort. "Hang on in their everyone we have raised the alarm and the firefighters will be there to get you out soon!" he warned.

Unfortunately, the confused lady Debra had proceeded to wet herself. "I know what we can do to get out we can all scream for attention I'll start' she began. It was then that Debra let out a blood-curdling deafening scream, she stopped and held her breath before letting out a loud scream.
"Right everyone please don't panic, when the ambulance team comes, we will be out of here in ten minutes but we have to be co-operative and quiet" John yelled.

Suddenly, disaster struck, and the bright lights in the lift faded to black, and the lift proceeded to crash down, becoming stuck again. I could feel the fear of the others in the lift, the sounds of heavy breathing and terror filled the room. "Is everybody ok?" John asked as he held his small flashlight out providing us all with a small speckle of light. "Oh yeah we are having a fantastic time, it's Monday morning, pitch black and I'm stuck in here." I yelled, "We'll get out of here if you want to leave no one's stopping you!" Debra gasped, growing more confused by the second. It was then that I switched on my phone, and I discovered I had over five missed calls, and a message from Sister Dana asking where I was. The ward was already short-staffed I couldn't imagine the damage my absence would have caused. Katie collapsed into a heap on the floor, breathing heavily. She explained that the experience of being locked in the lift brought her back to a time when she was locked in the toilet by bullies at school and was unable to leave for over two hours. Katie's breathing worsened and she ushered me to reach into her bag to get something, I found her inhaler and she used it, her hands were trembling, and her heavy breathing rate decreased.

The ambulance team arrived and we huddled together as they attempted to get us out. After five minutes the lift crashed down to the ground floor. Debra became increasingly confused and decided to stand up on the floor, and grabbed John by his neck, shouting, "You keeping us hostage let me out of here now," she pleaded. "Please Debra sit down, we will be out of here very soon," he warned. "I tell you what I will try I will scream see if they can hear me," "No!" Gabrielle shouted. It was then that Debra proceeded to scream continuously, forgetting she tried it earlier. I was struggling to keep my sanity in the lift between the awful protracted silences and the angry outbursts it was a terrifying situation. At 4 pm the firemen managed to release us from the lift. We were met by a crowd of hospital staff, firefighters and maintenance crews cheering us on. I quickly ran out of the lift and made my way home. I hope this was not a sign of what was to come. I arrived home and spent the afternoon in the hot tub watching the back to the future box set. I hoped I was able to successfully make the transition from student nurse to nurse.

CHAPTER 4: NURSING CHAOS

I returned to the stroke ward full of anticipation and fear, I avoided the lift and made sure I entered the ward early and that I was relaxed. I walked into the staff room, and I was greeted by Sister Dana who smiling and cheerful for the day ahead. The other nurse was called Elaine, a fifty-two-year-old nurse, with over thirty years of experience in the stroke ward. Then there was Helena a thirty-year-old nurse who worked part-time whilst studying for her masters in public health. Before the handover came, two student nurses, Beth and Lauren entered the ward. "Good morning girls, welcome to stroke ward B, your mentors will be Elaine and Helena," she smiled.

"Oh no I don't have students thank you, I've had enough of students!" Elaine scowled. I could feel myself starting to get angry, "You have not even met the students yet! It is your role as a nurse to mentor students you can't refuse!" I shouted. Elaine looked at me with anger and folded her arms in disgust.

It was then that I asked Dana about the men I looked after on the previous shift. Clive who suffered from dementia had moved to a dementia specialist care home, but the staff had rung the ward shortly after his visit explaining they were struggling with his unruly behavior.
David had moved to a specialist rehab facility, and made fantastic progress from being unable to mobilize, to mobilizing with a three-wheeled walker. Following my referral to the hospital mental health team, Liam had agreed to receive the counseling for his depression and was sent to an intermittent stroke rehab hospital to start his therapy program. It was then that my heart started to sink as Dana reported that Arnold passed away peacefully, the night I was locked in the lift. It was always difficult to accept that patients I cared for had passed, but I had to grow more resilient and to detach myself emotionally.

The night nurse Samantha arrived and handed over bay b, the female bay I would look after, including two women in the side rooms in the ward.
The first patient I was to look after was Ruth a 99-year-old confused lady at five foot four, who suffered a left-sided stroke and was admitted for further observation and an assessment after a fall at home. The second patient was a fifty-year-old lady called

Tina, who was admitted following a heart attack. Tina was a bank agency nurse at the hospital and I was warned that she had complained after every service and conversation she had.

The third patient was Trudy, a seventy nine-year-old lady who suffered a stroke and required full assistance with her personal care.

The first lady in the side room was Ethel an eighty-five-year-old lady who was admitted with diarrhea and vomiting and needed a side room to help prevent the spread of infection. The lady in the second room was Karen a 105-year-old lady, who worked as a typist in world war 2, she was admitted as an emergency patient with sepsis, but made a great recovery.

I worked alongside Sister Dana on the shift, as she overtook duties as my preceptor whilst disaster nurse Hayley was on holiday. Dana was an inspirational nurse, I watched as she introduced herself to the thirty patients in the ward. It was then that we completed the medication round, making sure that each patient took their required medication safely. I then worked alongside Dana to help wash the patients on the ward. We provided a bowl of water for Ruth and we pulled the curtain around her. Ruth looked very confused she sat in her bright pink nightgown, and her curly hair resembled a tower. "What are you up to? What is this bowl for?" Ruth then grabbed the bowl before throwing it on the floor. Dana

noticed Ruth's confused and asked her a number of questions, "Where are you?" she asked, "HMRC prison I suspect"
"What year is it"
"1922"
Dana became concerned at Ruth growing confusion, she explained to me how she was found wandering the streets with a shopping trolley, after leaving Tesco without paying for the items. Eventually, we managed to help Ruth with the wash, and as soon as we helped her to bed she fell asleep almost instantly.

We then proceeded to wash Trudy who had a full stroke. Trudy lay in her bed in her white nightdress with her blond wavy hair and bright blue eyes. Trudy had worked as a physiotherapist for over forty years and had lived an active life running competitively in local marathons. Around her bedside, Trudy had a range of photographs including a picture of her coming tenth in the London marathon, whilst another picture showed her standing proudly at her graduation with her parents, whilst another photo showed her about to jump off a plane for a skydive. she started to burst out crying, in the bed, "I'm sorry I just feel so hopeless, I'm so frightened, I've got so many plans and now this has happened," she sobbed. I held tightly onto Trudy's hand, "we are going to help you, Trudy, just work with us and participate in the therapy and remember we will take it day by day" I smiled. "Right Chris I just have to answer a call and attend the MDT meeting will you be ok for a second?" Dana asked. "Yes," I answered. I proceeded to prepare Trudy for a wash, and as I passed her a flannel. I felt a presence behind me. "How can I help," beamed the voice. It was Karen the 101-year-old patient in the side room who wanted to help us. Karen wore a blue apron and gloves. "It's ok Karen, we are managing fine." "Nonsense, I will help I mean I've made my bed, I'm going home tomorrow, and I need to get out of my room, You don't mind me helping you?" Karen asked Trudy. Trudy's wide-eyed confused expression spoke a thousand words. Thankfully Dana came along and helped Karen back to her room. We helped to wash Trudy and she required full assistance with turning in the bed and in washing. Trudy required full hoisting into her recliner chair.

As we drew the curtains an angry Tina sat in her bed in her white dressing gown and her arms folded in an angry stance. "Excuse me, I've been waiting for my morphine tablets all morning, I've pressed my buzzer this is not acceptable," she shouted. "OK Tina we will get your tablets but can we ask you to not shout at us please?" Dana pleaded. "I can shout if I like I'm the patient here, I can't wait to take my complaint to the health board!" she screeched. Tina was an example of a patient I had met on many other wards, a patient who would look to complain about anything she could find and gained great gratification in causing stress in others.

It was only 10 o'clock but already I was tired, working on the stroke ward was so physically demanding and I made sure I drank plenty of water but felt guilty if I sat down even for a second to rest.

I watched as Elaine walked past with her student Bethany, she was still miserable of the prospect to have to train a student. "Oh, Chris you need to go into side room one it looks like a bomb has gone off." Elaine smiled sarcastically. My heart started to sink, and as I walked into the side room I looked on in terror. Ethel sat in her armchair covered in poo, her colostomy bag had exploded and had spilled all over the floor and sprayed on the walls. "I'm so sorry I didn't realize how much of a mess I was in, but I tried to clean it up!" she gasped. I maintained a calm and relaxed composure when inside I wanted to scream! Thankfully Bethany saw me struggling as I wore my mask and gloves and began to mop the dirty floor. When we finished, Ethel looked up to me and took fifty pounds out of her purse, "I'm so sorry for what's happened, please accept this money as my apology," she smiled. "I can't take your money sadly but thank you!" I added.

At midday, at lunchtime, I helped mobilize the patients into wheelchairs and hospital chairs to participate in the singing group. The singing group was held in the therapy gym and was a revolutionary aspect of the nursing care the patients received. The stroke patients would sing familiar and old songs together. I watched in wonder after each session, as the music sessions helped the patients develop their speech, and helped to provide a stimulating cognitive activity to help them in their recovery process.

After the singing therapy session, Consultant Dr. Charles called me into the doctor's office for an important discussion. I instantly felt nervous in Dr. Charles present he had a very strict demeanor and wore a grey suit, with a red dicky bow, he wore thick black-rimmed glasses and had crazy wild black curly hair. Dr Charles gave me a stern look as he took a seat on his throne. "I have something to report to you, the scan results have come back for Trudy, she had a biopsy before her stroke. The results show she has cancer in her liver but it has spread throughout her body. Trudy's cancer is so advanced it's untreatable I have informed her," he groaned, before leaving the office.

I walked over to Trudy and she sat with her young daughter who was crying hysterically. I could feel tears roll down my cheek, I found it devastating that Trudy was already suffering after the stroke and now there was no hope for a full recovery. I placed my hand into Trudy's hand as the tears fell onto my hand. "If there is anything you want or need please don't hesitate to tell me," I nodded. "Is there anything that can help her? Any new chemotherapy we can try?" Marella her daughter asked. "Chemotherapy can only stabilize cancer in its present form at this stage, and attempt to slow the progression. We can have a conversation with Dr. Charles when he returns I added."

I wiped away my tears and had a break in the staffroom, it was the hardest part of being a nurse being unable to help people in their time of weakness, but it was an honor to look after people in their darkest hours.

My break was only half an hour long but I felt refreshed after eating my pasta bake and chocolate cake slice. When I returned to the ward area I had a range of tasks to complete, including taking notes, completing a medication round, and completing the end of bed notes, to keep a record of the patient's observations.

As I walked out of the staffroom Dana called us in for our staff huddle, which was completed at 1 pm each day. The staff huddle gave us a great opportunity as a team to discuss the patients in our bays, and to discuss any concerns that we had. Dana had prepared twenty pieces of buttered slices of toast for us, and a cup of tea for each member of staff. I observed the new students remembering that I was in their position three months prior to gaining the position. Bethany was enthusiastic and recorded notes in her notebook and was eager to learn new skills. Lauren, however, seemed to take a laid back approach, she arrived back from her lunch ten minutes late, constantly started to text her friends at the nurse's station. I wanted to intervene to help her before she would feel Elaine's wrath.

I started to complete the patient observations and firstly took Karen's observations. When I walked into the room, she was sitting in her armchair knitting a Christmas jumper. I admired her strength at the age of 105 she was independently mobile, completing her shopping independently, and going to church, and attending acting lessons on a weekly basis. Karen had a backpack and was waiting for her medications to be discharged. I delegated for the healthcare Juba to take Elaine for her scan. It felt wonderful to have the power to delegate jobs, without asking for permission from my mentor.

Suddenly Dana let out a terrifying scream, "Chris quick it's Rita!" she panicked. I ran into the bay and felt my heart skip a beat in a state of nervousness. I looked on in Shock Rita Was laying on the floor arms outstretched on her covers. Rita had ripped the blue curtains off the curtain rail and knocked down all the items on her table. "Get me out of here now I want to go home!" she screamed. It was then that I helped Dana to hoist Rita back into her armchair. I had to request for Marsha the healthcare assistant to provide one to one assistance to Rita as she was at a high risk of falling. It was one of the greatest challenges of working on a ward, supervising a confused patient, whilst trying to meet the needs of all the patients in my care.

Ten minutes later I was notified that Ethel's scan results were clear and she was ready to be discharged alongside Karen. The ambulance arrived quickly, there were five stroke patients in the a and e department and the ward was pushing for discharges. As I peered into Side room two I witnessed Karen dressed in a floral dress, with large brown oversized sunglasses and she carried her brown satchel. "If you ever require any volunteers to help out please give me a ring, I'd be happy to help, you have all been like a family to me!" she beamed. I marveled at her strength and her burst of energy at 105!

It was then that my two new patients were admitted. The first patient was Sheena Bladavoia a patient who was unable to speak English and had only recently moved to England from India two days ago. Sheena entered the ward with her Son Rashid and daughter Shauna, who were able to translate for her. Sheen was four foot five and wore a long white dress, her hair was long and flowed down to her feet. Shauna was admitted following recurrent headaches and was suspected of having a TIA stroke. "Mother would like four towels, a tea with four sugars, six pillows and five blankets," sauna smiled. I took Sheena's observation and found that her temperature was over forty degrees, her heart rate and respirations were of a high rate, which means that she succeeded the threshold and required support from the critical care team. I could see that Sheena was in pain and she began to sweat excessively.

The second patient to arrive was Matthew Clarke a seventy nine-year-old man who was admitted due to his unstable diabetic readings, with a past history of a left-sided stroke. He waltzed in the ward with his walking stick, angrily with his wife in the room. "Hello Matthew I'm Chris I am a nurse who will be looking after you today, can I take your observations? I asked. Matthew proceeded to kick the observation machine out of the way, angrily, "No please, I just want to go home, I was sent to A and E, by my GP, overreacting but I can't stay!" he growled. "We need to monitor your diabetic readings," I added. "Just get your manager I've got shoes older than you, and no offense but I don't take advice from a child," he shouted.

It was dinner time and chaos had erupted in my bay, Rita began to throw Items from her table across the bay as her confusion worsened. Rita wanted to make a complaint about the healthcare Marsha who she believed was texting on her phone. Trudy's family was requesting her to be moved to a side room due to the high level of noise in the bay. Then I looked at the corner of the room, and Sheena had her blue curtain drawn around her, as I peered in I looked on in shock over thirty members of her family were there including her seven siblings, five children, and ten young grandchildren. Then Mr. Clarke stormed into the room, "I'm sorry there are far too many people here, only two people per patient, please leave!" he stammered. When Mr. Clarke assessed Sheena he believed she had a bacterial infection and he prescribed her with paracetamol intravenously.

Luckily I was able to get support with Dana who helped me to maintain a calm atmosphere in the ward, making sure the patients were settled for bed. My final task was completing a diabetic checklist, I discovered that Matthew was drinking alcohol excessively each day, and had a box in his bedroom filled with a dozen chocolate bars that he would constantly refill. I referred Matthew to the diabetic specialist nurse to help him to manage his poorly treated condition.

CHAPTER 5: NURSING ON THE FRONT LINE.

It was a bright, warm, Sunday morning I woke up to the sounds of the bluebirds chirping in the oak trees. One of the reasons I loved living in Yorkshire was the peace and quiet I felt. In my apartment in New York, I could constantly hear the sound of car horns beeping, people passing by shouting, and bright lights flashing through the blinds.

I made myself a warm cup of tea and had my porridge with golden syrup. I felt so happy and relaxed working on the stroke ward at the weekend was usually a more relaxed pace. I didn't realize how wrong I could be, I was about to face my hardest shift as a qualified nurse.

I entered the staff room at 7 am, Sister Dana sat at the table with the handover sheets ready to distribute. Sitting next to Dana were the healthcare assistants Sara and Becky. "Chris I am sorry to tell you but Nurse Cathy and nurse Emilia have called in sick. I have informed the hospital management team and they are trying to send extra staff to the ward."
I could feel my heart start to sink, with three members of staff off sick it made our working day more challenging.

"Sister Dana, how are we going to cope? Thirty patients and two nurses we will never do it!" I warned.

"I have a plan, instead of working separately we will work as a team, Becky and Sara will work together to complete the ward washes, we will complete the drug round together, and then join in with them!" she began, her face glowing red with fear.
When I walked onto the ward I witnessed the devastating impact that short staff levels can have on a ward environment. We were desperately running around, making sure each patient was sat up and had adequate food to eat. Helping patients with their food took an extra half an hour on the shift.

I worked together with Dana to complete the drug round, during this round we had to help patients to the toilet, change a patient's pad, and admit a new patient on the ward. Without the correct staffing levels, we were put under enormous pressure to keep the patients safe. The phone rang and Dana answered it, it was the hospital team explaining that two staff members from another department had refused to be moved to the stroke ward, but they were attempting to get more staff.

During the end of the ward round, an elderly confused patient called Daniel was attempting to escape the ward, using his walking as an attempt to break down the door. He stood by the door, angry, in his green pajamas with his pants over the trousers. "Let me out he shouted, Let me out or so help me God I will smash my way out," he shouted. I calmly walked over to Daniel "Can you walk with me back to your bed space, I can make you a cup of tea." I offered. It was then that Daniel flew into a deep rage, I ducked as he attempted to hit me with his walking stick, smashing the nurses' station. Suddenly he grabbed my hand and began to bite into it. Dana arrived and suddenly his mood changed, her relaxed composure and distraction technique helped to carm Daniel's behavior. "Daniel take a walk with me to the garden, we can have a nice chat there and you can help name the different birds you can see." She smiled. Dana had a very calm and relaxed nature, and was instantly able to relax patients when they were distressed.

When Dana arrived back we joined Becky and Sara and helped to complete the morning washes. Together we helped to wash fifteen patients, we hoisted patients into a chair and made sure that each patient was safe and comfortable.
By 12am we were exhausted and ready to sleep. The hospital bed manager had managed to recruit another nurse to take over a bay, and a healthcare assistant called Shelley to give Daniel one to one support. Our nursing staff levels were safe but only just. In a stroke of good luck, we managed to discharge fifteen patients that day leaving fifteen patients on the ward.

I was looking after five patients in my bay, including Daniel who was now sleeping in his bed. The other patients included Jake a seventeen-year-old boy with autism who was suffering from seizures. Jake's mum was a nightmare complaining about every aspect of his care.

The next patient was Matthew a thirty-nine- year- old man who was admitted with a stroke and refused to get involved with the therapy team in order to aid his recovery. Micheal had been reported by staff for smoking and eating junk food, that his family sneaked in for him, entirely against the doctor's orders.

Then the next patients were Garry and Steven. Garry was an eighty-five year- old man admitted following recurrent TIA's whilst Steven was admitted as a social admission having struggled with depression and anxiety, following the death of his wife three years later. Steven's sister had phoned the ambulance when she went round to visit him, he had fallen down the stairs and his house was in a terrible condition.

Garry and Steven became close friends and were often seeing playing charades and competing against each other with the daily newspaper crosswords. They were the perfect patients.

I continued through my shift, I wondered how I survived the morning, but could not have succeeded without Dana who displayed calmness in spite of the difficulties we faced.

At 3 pm I started to complete my ward round notes when Jake's mum Claudine, stomped towards me in her platform shoes, her beady green eyes glared into mine, as her blonde hair towered over her like Marge Simpson. "I am not happy with the care of my son, his lunch was cold! You have no air conditioning on the ward and you're short-staffed, ohh I can't wait to speak to your manager!" she shouted, her face turning bright red in anger. Claudine continued to shout at me I pretend to listen but instead, I was thinking of the song 'raining in my heart' by Buddy Holly as I watched the rain poured down outside. I had come across aggressive relatives before, and even though I was providing the best care I could give for her son, she continued to complain about anything and everything.

I walked over to Dana who was sitting at the nurses' station, "Thank you for your help this morning," I beamed. "It's fine we worked together as a team, hopefully, our recruitment drive next week will bring more new staff to the ward. In the meantime I want you to check Matthew's bedside to see if he's been hiding any junk food or any drug paraphernalia please," she ushered.

I walked over to mIcheals bed space, he had the curtains drawn around him, as I peered through I watched him laying on the bed in his black tracksuit eating his Mcdonald's. I slowly crept in, "Matthew try to keep to the diet that Dr. Ray put you on," I offered. "Excuse me, please don't tell me what to do you child, I can do what I want, go away!" he screeched, throwing the food waste at me I looked around the space and found rolled up cigarettes on the floor, and realized that I had to report this to sister Dana and that he would require one to one supervision.

At 4 pm Shelley went on her break and I had to take over care of Daniel.
Daniel used to be a doctor and spent most of his time writing on his notepad believing he was still working as a GP. As soon as I sat next to Micheal he instantly became agitated. "I thought I told you to keep away from me!" he stammered. "I'm here to look after you," I replied.
"No I have to go I have to be at the GP surgery for 9 am tomorrow." he scowled. Daniel proceeded to stand up grabbing his stick. As he walked towards the main door Dana instantly grabbed Daniel by his hands, and let Daniel into a waltz. I watched in awe as they danced happily through the ward. I always admired Dana as a manager, she was Carm, patient and had a great sense of humor.

My time on the stroke was was invaluable, the majority of staff worked together to improve patient care, and most importantly the management team supported staff wellbeing at all times. I learned how to look after patients who suffered from a stroke and required emergency care, and how to support patients with their journey in regaining their mobility.

On the night after my final shift, I arrived home, unaware of what I was going to face, and I was not prepared for what was to come. I was reflecting on what had happened over the past year and went into my brother's room trying to come to terms with his death, putting his items in boxes, something I had avoided.

It was so difficult looking through Michael's boxes I felt like I was intruding on his private information. Even though Michael was my twin he kept his life as a doctor private, and whilst he attended University in Belfast for five years, I only saw him once a month and during the Christmas break.

I felt very emotional looking through the boxes of diaries, clothes, and pictures he kept hidden. As I looked through his diary he kept as a student doctor I discovered he faced his own troubles, anxiety, and fear of the possibility of failing his exams, and the constant pressure of completing practical skills under constant scrutiny left him struggling to sleep at night. I also discovered in Michael's diary that he was in a serious relationship with a girl named Susan, but the relationship broke down when she decided to exit the course and move back to Scotland. I was seeing a different side to Michael, the side he kept fiercely private. Our final years together included trips to the beach, nights at the movies, and taking long bike rides together, but Michael's time at university was always a mystery to all of us.

I spent the evening watching the sunset whilst sitting on the garden patio when suddenly I heard a knock on the door. I had been on my own for three months, and my parents were due back later in the year. I opened the door to a young lady at twenty-six carrying a small child around 4 years of age. The young woman was beautiful with glowing skin and bright blue ocean colored eyes. The little boy resembled his mum in looks but also looked familiar to me, it was as if I had met him before. "Hi I'm Susan I'm looking for Michael, I believe this his address?" she asked looking at me startled. "You must be Chris, you're practically Michael's double!" She beamed. I looked on at Susan nervously. "Please come in," I smiled, walking the mysterious woman and her child into the dining room.

I quickly realized that Susan was the woman Michael had been writing about. I explained that Michael had passed away, and Susan began to break down in shock and stated that she felt enormous guilt, knowing that she never told him that he had a son, the little boy was Michael's child. I looked at him as he sat in my Father's rocking chair holding his train set. Thomas had the same hair eye color and smile as Michael.

"I'm so sorry, I'm in shock, I just wish he knew, I see Michael in your son in my nephew!" I smiled. I walked into the kitchen to make Susan a warm hot chocolate, and by the time I walked back into the room, she had left the house, whilst leaving her number on the dining room table.

I felt myself reeling, trying to absorb the fact that I was an uncle, and imagined how different Michael's life may have been if he had met his son.

CHAPTER 6: THE MEDICAL WARD

I was nervous on the first day of my second rotation in a general medical ward. I felt so supported in the stroke ward, I could turn to any staff member and I would be helped straight away.

I arrived at the medical ward at 7 am for the handover in a small cluttered staffroom with a widescreen television. I was surrounded by five staff members. The sister Lucy was a newly qualified nurse at twenty-six and was leading the handover, she refused to look me in the eyes, only glancing at me quickly. The second nurse was Belsida who had thirty years of experience as a nurse and had previously completed her training in the Philippines, she smiled and held onto my trembling knee to offer me comfort. The third nurse was Greg a twenty-two-year-old nurse who looked exhausted as he began to clench his fists. Louisa and Hannah were the healthcare assistants on the shift. I instantly missed the staff on the stroke ward, especially Dana who provided me the most support.

It was then that the night nurse handed over my patients for the shift. My first patient was Sophie an eighty-five-year-old lady with the early stages of dementia. Sophie was admitted as a social admission as paramedics bought in after setting her kitchen on fire whilst attempting to cook a turkey dinner.

In the second side room was a twenty-five-year-old man Joseph who was admitted following a suicide attempt at home, and was admitted to the hospital after attempting to hang himself to a tree in his garden.

Then the nurse introduced the five patients in my bay. The first man was Erick a ninety-year-old man with dementia, admitted due to a nursing home stating they struggled to look after him due to his aggressive behavior.

The second patient was Gareth, a thirty-five-year-old man admitted for excessive alcohol consumption, and was undertaking a detox program.

The third patient was Sean a fifty-six-year-old man admitted after being found wandering on the motorway in the middle of the night.

The fourth patient was Jeremy seventy nine-year-old man admitted for investigation after experiencing recurrent headaches.

The fifth patient was Simon an eighty-two-year-old man who had tried to cope with his dementia illness on his own, but he was arrested after throwing items around in a local supermarket and attacking a check out assistant. After further investigation, he was diagnosed with Lewy body dementia.

I felt nervous as I began to complete my medication round. I was on my own in a ward where the staff appeared hostile. I walked around the ward and noticed that the ward was painted with dementia-friendly pastel colors, and the clocks had a picture of the sun to show it was daytime, whilst the moon picture would replace the sun at 7 pm.

I walked around my bay and I realized I was being faced with challenges already. Eric had thrown his porridge on the floor and smashed the plate. Sean was wandering around the bay in his white dressing gown, hallucinating trying to climb a ladder he believed he could see by the window.

The other men in the bay were asleep, as were the patients in the side room. I completed my medication rounds with ease, whilst I completed the rounds Louisa and Hannah hoisted Eric behind the curtains into the armchair. I could hear him kicking and screaming, as they made him comfortable in the recliner chair before they hurried off to help the other nurses. I gave Jeremy, Simon, Sean and Gareth bowls so they could have a wash.

Suddenly Etic became more aggressive trying to get out of the chair. I walked out of the bay calling for help, The health care assistant explained they were too busy to help, whilst Sister Lucy said she would try to help after her meeting. I started to get frustrated and grabbed the phone from the nurse's station, and called the charge nurse who luckily managed to move a health care assistant from another ward to sit with Eric. Etic began to hit out at me and Sara and with a great struggle, we managed to change his incontinence pad to make him feel comfortable.

I asked through the blue curtains if the men required any assistance with their wash. "I'm finished!" shouted Simon. As I walked in I looked on in shock as Simon mistook his net pants as a t-shirt and attempted to put his hand through them, I helped to support him with getting changed and wondered how he managed to live on his own. I checked on the other patients who had managed to wash independently. I provided Gareth with a blanket as he began to shiver. He was thankful for being on the alcohol detox program, and finally getting medical treatment. Gareth's excessive drinking over a twenty-year period had cost him his wife and children and home.

Once my patients in the bay were ready for the day ahead I walked into the side room to check on Sophie. As I walked into the room Sophie was lying in her bed with a Cinderella bedspread, and her nightlight light projected images of farmyard animals on the wall. In the cot was the fake baby she believed was hers. Sophie was diagnosed with early-stage dementia but was also suffering from Schizophrenia and severe autism. She looked confused in the bed she looked at me with her bright blue eyes and wild curly hair. "Good morning Sophie I wanted to ask you if you were ready for a wash this morning?" "Go away get out of my house!" she whispered. "This is not your home your in a side room on a hospital ward," I added. "Shhh you'll wake the baby!" she whispered sternly. I walked over the lifelike doll in the cot. The doll looked creepy and grotesque features, bright red hair, and piercing creepy green eyes that peered into mine. The doll had a battery pack attached which enabled the doll to breathe. Suddenly the doll's expression changed and it burst out crying. "Oh dear Please pass me, my baby," Sophie pleaded. I went to put my hands in the cot, accidentally kicking the wooden stand, causing the cot to break and the baby to roll on the floor. Suddenly Sophie jumped out of the bed screaming, "My baby my baby you've killed it you bastard!" she shouted. Sophie then pushed me against the wall before hitting me across the face.

Then nurse Blesida appeared behind me, grabbing Sophie's hand, "C'mon Sophie I have your baby now, I will protect her," she smiled. Blesida offered to help Sophie with a wash, she turned to me and smiled, "I know the staff seem unfriendly at the start but they are just wary of new staff you will settle in no time!" she smiled. Blesida's Kind words made such a difference, it only took one person's kind words to make me feel settled.

I walked into the second side room to check on Joseph. Joseph sat in his blue tracksuit, crying on his bed, pulling his hair in frustration. I grabbed a chair and sat next to him. "I'm here to help you today if there is anything you need please let me know," I offered. "How long have you felt depressed for?" I asked. "Six months ago I was driving my car with my girlfriend and best friend Mark. It was a beautiful hot day, and we were singing on the long drive down the motorway. I dropped my phone when I dropped it I lost control of my car and crashed into a family of three in another car, they all died including Mark and Abby, I was the only survivor." he cried. "I'm so sorry, there is so much support out there for you the hospital has a wonderful counseling service and I am here to help you," I added.
"I just feel like the guilt is too much and the grieving process never ends," he added. As I looked on at his face he appeared so lost and afraid. I could see myself in him when I was grieving for Michael, I felt so hopeless and I empathize with him. I referred Joseph for an urgent meeting with the hospital's rapid response mental health team to speak about local support for him. I wanted to talk further with him to offer support but I had to complete my assigned tasks and end of bed paperwork. I always felt as a student I never had as much time as I would like to talk to patients, as the pressure of not completing the paperwork accurately weighed heavy on my shoulders.

I took my morning break in the bland hospital cafeteria with shepherds pie and chocolate cake on the walls. I sat down to eat my cold pasta and cheese, as I looked up I saw my previous nursing school classmate Clive. Clive was working as a nurse practitioner in the A and E apartment, he came across very arrogant and often took over conversations with his own egotistical beliefs. "Hey, Chris how are you doing?" he asked "well-" I'm working in A and E I'm a senior mentor to students, and it looks like I'm on the top of the list for a promotion! I heard you joined a small theatre group," he sneered.

I started to daydream nodding to what he was saying. I thought about my time as an actor in New York, the rave reviews, the rapturous applause from the crowd, and the support from colleagues. As a nurse, I felt undervalued and scrutinized over every task, but seeing the patients make good outcomes made the job so worthwhile.

I returned from my break and took over the supervision of Eric whilst Isabelle went on her break. Erick's wife stood in her blue coat and held her green purse across her chest, her hair was pink and wrapped in silver curlers. " Eric you're wife's here to see you," I said, softly leaning in closer. Eric sat angrily in his green pajamas with his fingers clenched, his face was boiling red. "That woman over there is not my wife she's my Grandmother Bertie and I hate her!" He stammered. Part of Eric's dementia illness made him believe that he was a child, and he had no recollection of his adult life. I tried to devise a way to engage Eric with his wife and I put the radio on and the Elvis song, 'can't help falling in love' started to play. I immediately noticed a change in Eric he began to relax and really concentrated, as he listening to the lyrics, "Oh Mary we use to love this song, we use to dance to it at the church hall!" Eric smiled. Mary moved closer and held onto Eric's hand as she began to cry. I learned as a trainee nurse the powerful effect music had on the brain, and how songs can help patients with dementia positively reminisce about the past.

I then had to complete my daily tasks making sure that the daily charts such as fluid and food intake were filled in. It was then that I witnessed Gareth visibly shaking in his armchair, I walked over to him trying to find he was slurring his speech and appeared confused, his eyes were widening, and he could not talk. It was my first emergency as a qualified nurse and I panicked. I could tell he was showing symptoms of a hypo, as he was diabetic, and when I took his blood sugar reading I discovered that his reading was abnormally low.

I quickly ran for the diabetes crash box which contained the glucagon tablets and glucagon gel. When I walked back to the chair, I put on the nursing gloves and rubbed the glucagon gel on Gareth's gums. Gareth began to sweat profusely in the chair and had knocked the contents of his books and food on his table on the floor. After a few minutes, and after Gareth had the glucagon tablets I noticed a rapid change, his breathing became more controlled, and he started to become more oriented to time and place. I had arranged for the social worker to see Gareth, to provide support on his living situation, as he wanted to gain supervised access to his daughter, and I booked Gareth to have a meeting with the ward's designated mental health team to help with his depression.

I then had to complete my second test of the day to complete a mocha test, a mini-mental health test to check Sean's cognition and to test for a possible link towards dementia. The test tested cognition, memory call, numeracy, comprehension, and orientation. The test included a practical test in which Sean would have to draw a clock face with the correct symbols and a 3-d box. I went through the questions with Sean, he showed he was disoriented as he believed the year was 1983 and that he was in a hospital in London. I gave Sean three words apple, goat, and pig, five minutes later he was unable to recall the words. Sean was unable to complete the basic numeracy calculations, or draw a clock face. He scored one out of twenty-seven for the mental health test.

The ward doctor explained he had never seen a score so slow for a man in his early 50's and on further consultation with the doctor, he referred him to the memory clinic for suspected dementia. It was devastating to see how confused and unstable Sean was. In the morning his sister Trudy arrived explained that he was a dentist for twenty-five years, and took early retirement, as he was planning to travel the world. It always shocked me how fast dementia could progress. As a student I watched people in the hospital grow more and more confused during their hospital stay, as many patients presented with delirium.

Dr. Clive had called me into a meeting in the nurse's office with Jeremy the patient who had suffered recurrent headaches and his wife who sat wearing her bright blue summer dress, with bright blue oversized sunglasses. Dr. Clive sat he appeared concerned, his glasses sat at the bottom of his nose, and his face contorted to worry. "Mr. and Mrs. Kettering, I have the results of Gareth's scan here," he mumbled. "Oh doctor I'm so glad that Gareth is finally in hospital, ever since he has had the headaches, he has angry outbursts, he is depressed, he's become more and more disoriented," she murmured, her hands started to tremble, and tears rolled down her cheek in anticipation for the news.

"Gareth I am very sorry to have to tell you, but the scan showed multiple Mets and you have a tumor in your brain which can not be removed," he added, robotically, as he clenched further onto the scan results of the brain. "There must be something you can do, some kind of wonder drug, there must be!" she pleaded. "I'm very sorry but this type of cancer is untreatable, we can start you on a course of chemotherapy to delay the spread of cancer," he said sternly. I then sat and watched as Mrs. Kettery collapsed into Mr. Kettering's arms.

Suddenly I was transported back to when my own brother Michael was in the doctor's office and found that he had a grade 4 brain tumor. At first, I started to think irrationally and contemplated sending him to America to try an experimental form of chemotherapy, and to try the latest liquid diets that were believed to cure cancer. I was in denial, refusing to accept that my brother's condition was terminal. I remember the shock on his face, he was numb, it was almost like an explosion had occurred in the room. I started to cry along with Gareth and his wife, being in the same situation again sent shivers through me. I watched as Gareth and his wife returned to his bedside. They talked about a range of topics ranging from chemotherapy, to how they were going to inform key members of the family.

Then nurse Blesida explained that she was going on her break, and asked me to keep an eye on her patients in her bay. Bles had only three patients in the bay and had managed to discharge three patients previously. The patients included a forty-five-year-old lady called Hayley, who had been admitted for heart surgery for a valve replacement, Shelia a lady admitted following a worsening in her MS condition, and Jill who was admitted following a history of struggling to manage her type 2 diabetes condition.

Hayley was mewsing a seven which meant her heart rate respiration rate and blood pressure were above the normal parameters. Blesida had put her on five liters of oxygen and she was due to have observations every fifteen minutes. I watched as she lay on top of the covers in her red dressing gown, her face was pale, but she managed to smile as she grabbed onto my hand, "Please nurse can you call my daughters to come and see me? She whispered.

I called Hayley's daughter following her request but I grew concerned as I walked past the side room, I noticed that Joseph had barricaded himself in the side room and had locked himself in the bathroom. I called the security and they arrived on the ward and helped me to open the main door, and they used a spanner to open the bathroom door. We walked in just in time, as Joseph had tied his white bed sheet around his neck and had attempted to hang himself in the bathroom. I helped him down unraveling the linen from around his neck and I helped him to the bathroom floor where he broke down crying in a flood of tears.
"Joseph I'm going to get a member of the mental health team to sit with you for a while, I want you to accept our help, you have so much to live for," I added. I felt so worried for Joseph he was struggling with post-traumatic stress disorder. In his mind, Joseph was

struggling to come to terms with the car accident and had kept his trauma hidden.

My shift on the medical ward had been so difficult, I missed the strong team ethic of the staff on the stroke ward, the staff on the medical ward were so hostile, I realized how important it was to be part of a strong team. Just as I entered my bay I heard the emergency siren begin to ring out, it was like a fog horn ringing out. I could feel the surge of adrenaline running through me, my heart pounded against my chest. The emergency buzzer rang from nurse Blesida's bay, from Hayley, who had gone into cardiac arrest. I rushed towards her space and began to complete the thirty compressions.

Suddenly a stampede of doctors nurses and health care assistants surrounded Hayley. The crash trolley had arrived, and the senior CPR advance nurse had entered the ward. As I completed the compressions I could feel my arms start to ache, and I began to sweat with fear, breathing into the air mask, desperately trying to revive Hayley, I wanted her to respond, she wanted to see her daughters. It was then that the senior doctor took over the compressions, but there was no response. The compressions lasted for over fifteen minutes, and finally, Sister Lucy used the defibrillator but Hayley was pronounced dead at 5pm. It was so difficult watching Hayley's daughters arrive in their woolly jackets, expecting to see her before Bles took them into the nurse's office to break the bad news.

I walked into my bay and took a seat next to Eric who was still holding hands with his wife Mary. Mary looked over to me smiling. "Thank you for helping us and for guiding me to find the best care home for Eric. It has been so difficult for both of us to agree to what is the best in terms of his care but you have really helped," she murmured.

I made sure I completed all of the tasks I needed to fulfill in my shift. In conjunction with the social worker, I found the right care for Eric. Sophie had been referred for counseling, and I booked for her to meet with Ica care psychiatric unit which would help her intermittently until her mood had stabled. I organized a one to one mental health nurse to supervise Joseph at all times, and he had booked to enter a private local wellbeing rehab center to help him to come to terms with the tragic events he faced. I arranged a multidisciplinary team to talk about Gareth's detox program and to review his medication. I arranged for Sean to have a brain scan and a further consultation with the doctor to check for dementia. I organized for Jeremy to receive palliative care at home, and for nurses to see him three days a week, to provide emotional and physical support. I had organized for Simon to be seen by the nursing discharge team and social worker to find him a suitable place to live.

My time on the medical ward was very difficult. The morale in the ward was very low, and the staff were not supported by the senior members of the nursing team. Many of the newly qualified nurses had left the ward after six months, I felt as if I was surviving in my role rather than exceeding in my role. I felt in my second rotation I was still finding my feet as a qualified nurse. I had participated in ward emergencies, managed the care of critically ill patients, and achieved proficiency in my basic nursing skills. At times I wanted to run to a 'mentor' to get the emotional support I needed, but I was on my own.

CHAPTER 7: HOLIDAY

It was time for my winter's break in Northumberland at my parent's
cottage where I was to be reunited with my parents after a year's
break. I had not informed my parents yet of my decision to complete my newly qualified year as a nurse after my successful year
as an actor. I worried about what my parents would say. Since my
brother had passed away I felt I was trying to please everyone.
I had put so much effort into my nursing course over the three

years, I wanted to complete a year working as a nurse to apply the knowledge I learned, without living a life of regret wondering what it would be like to be a nurse on the front line.

The cottage in Northumberland was full of family memories, situated right next to boulmer beach in Alnwick. As a child I would play badminton with my brother on the beach, we would jump off the cliff edge and swim in the crystal blue ocean sea, and in the afternoons we would sit around my Grandfather's grand piano, with the warm fire burning. After my brother passed away he had renovated the cottage filled with old family photos, and new furniture.

When I arrived at the cottage it was a beautiful summer day. I took a morning swim in the ocean and spent the evening looking through old family photos. I then lay on the deck chair on the garden patio, listening to the crash of the waves against the ocean. I felt so relaxed, for the first time in two years.

At 8 pm my parents arrived, and my mother embraced me after not seeing me for a whole year, following their stay in California. My mother had aged so much in the year following the death of my brother. Her brown her was now curly and grey, her complexion was pale, and her eyes made her look so lost and alone.
"It's so wonderful to see you! What have you been doing since you arrived home? You have to remember to keep up to date with the acting agency, just in case they have another role lined up to you," Mum smiled.
I've taken a role as a rotational band five nice at a Yorkshire trust, I'm six months into my rotation, and I'm going into a community setting soon." I took a deep breath as I could see my parents reeling from the shock of what I revealed.

"You're going to throw your acting career away! The money you made from the shows set you up for the future you can't just walk away from it! Nursing was not for you!" she shouted.

"It's just something I have to do!" I added.

I noticed the anger on my parent's face, they were so invested in me becoming an actor, but nursing was allowing me to be around people and helped to curb the loneliness I felt.

My holiday in Northumberland with my parents was spent reminiscing about the past, taking long bike rides in the countryside in the morning, playing badminton on the beach, and redecorating the guest rooms upstairs. We arrived back in Yorkshire on Sunday the 1st of September the day before I was to start on my third rotation. I was to work in the community in a pilot telephone service which aimed to help the elderly who suffered from falls, and were diagnosed with dementia, through advice and practical support.

Before I went to sleep that night I noticed a red-letter addressed to me, that had been posted whilst we were away. It was in my twin brother Michael's handwriting. On the front, it read 'to be opened on 2nd of February' in what was to be my 28th Birthday. I wondered what Michael had planned what message he had sent. Since he passed he left several messages and surprises for us. Michael had left me his money in his will and his car, he pre-recorded video requesting me to follow my dream to become an actor, and he reunited my sister to our family through a letter he sent. The letters he had prepared made it harder to let him go, but they felt like he was still communicating with us, and that made them even more special. I took the envelope upstairs and locked it away in my cupboard.

CHAPTER 8: NURSING TELEPHONE SERVICE

I woke up on a cold Monday morning, waiting to start my third nursing rotation in the community as part of a pilot nursing service. The telephone service was created to support elderly people who had experienced falls, been discharged from hospital, and were living with conditions such as dementia.

It was such a different environment working in the telephone service. When I arrived at the small cabin office it was a world away from life on the wards. The office had twenty desks each with a computer and phone set. The team was made of sixteen nurses, a physiotherapist, and two nursing supervisors. I had to take a training course with four other new starters. Through role-play and online training courses we learned how to respond to adults in emergencies over the phone, and how to assess the home environment. The job included making both outgoing and incoming calls to patients discharged from the hospital. In the afternoons we were each assigned a caseload of patients to visit at their homes.

Callers rang for many different reasons, including helping with completing activities at home, support with medication, and crisis support for carers looking after relatives at home. At times we would receive phone calls from people who required counseling for emotional support.

On my first day I was greeted by three other nurses who were starting the same day as me. Jenny was a fifty-five-year-old nurse with over thirty years as a community district nurse and was very ill-tempered and angry. Louisa was a twenty four-year-old nurse, she constantly sang in the office, often distracting the other staff. Maria was a sixty-year-old nurse, and was six foot five, and believed that she was a fountain of knowledge, constantly demeaning other staff.

I was so nervous as I sat at my office desk on the first day, I looked at the other nurses chatting away on the phone, the clicking of the keyboard, the ringing of the phone, I was not used to sitting down, I almost felt a sense of guilt.

Suddenly the phone started to ring, "Hello I'm Chris Nurse Together, how can I help you?"
"Can I have a chicken tikka masala, boiled rice, poppadoms, and two nans bread?" said the caller.
"I'm sorry this is a nursing service you have the wrong number," I added before the caller hung up. I began to panic, hoping that I

was not going to get any more inappropriate calls, my heart was still racing with nervous adrenaline running through me.

I then received my second call from a lady called Deborah with dementia who had rung as an emergency call.

"Hello, Chris nurse together how can I help you?"
"Hi this is Deborah, I'm calling because I need some help, carers have gone but I need the toilet, and I have pains in my chest, I can't get up from my armchair," She cried, her shrill voice echoing through the phone. "Is there anyone you can ring? A family member?" I asked. "I have my son's phone number in my phonebook here,"
"Can I have it?" I asked.
I could hear Deborah breathing heavily, she appeared anxious and worried. "Right the number is 01ptt7t....." Deborah's dementia had affected her ability to read coherently. "I live Glestown avenue number 6," she stated. It was then that she stood up from her armchair, "I need to answer the doorbell," she whispered, Suddenly I could hear a loud thud Deborah took a loud fall onto a wooden floor. I could hear her crying out in pain, "Deborah can you hear me? Are you there? Oh, Deborah please tell me!" I pleaded. I immediately rang the ambulance, I could picture Deborah laying helplessly on the floor, I feared she was injured, I wanted to physically help her. The barrier of being behind a phone hit me, I was limited as to what I could do.

It was so distressing knowing that I could not physically help her, there was no time to reflect as the phone started to ring.

"Hello, Chris I am Stella, I need some help my husband keeps on having falls in the house and in the garden, yesterday, he took a fall down four steps of the garden patio," she cried. "How is your husband now?" I asked. "He is settled now, but he is struggling to mobilize only short distances around the house, I can't cope, can you please send a nurse and physiotherapist to the house to assess him?" She cried hysterically reaching for help. I logged her referral to the physiotherapist, but again I found it distressing listening to her difficult situation on the phone.

I looked around the room to find the nurses typing away, whispering, and scribbling away at their notepads. I felt very nervous having spent so many years on the wards, and it felt so nerve-wracking sitting down at the desk. On the wards, it was easier to communicate with patients once I was given a handover. On the phones, I was unprepared and having to think of outcomes quickly for the clients.

The phone started to ring again, "Chris nurse together how can I help you?" I asked.
"I'm Eileen I'm ringing looking for some help, I'm sorry I have to whisper, it's just my husband is asleep and he has dementia, and he gets paranoid when I'm on the phone. For weeks his condition has declined, last weekend we went to the supermarket, and he was kicked out for throwing items off the conveyor belt, and hitting the shopkeeper with a tin of beans."

"Does your husband have carers in place?" I asked. It was then that I could hear Eileen crying hysterically on the phone.
"I have been trying to cope on my own but life is getting so difficult, he swears at me constantly, he is always arguing with me, and last night he smashed two of the windows in the bathroom. I'm also struggling because he keeps falling throughout the house! Please help me I can't cope!" she cried.

"Eileen try and take a deep breath and remain calm. I was wondering if it is possible to visit your house this afternoon with our trained physiotherapist to assess your husband?"
"That would be so helpful thank you!" she explained. I could hear the nervousness in her voice, as a carer she had hit crisis point and required urgent help.

It was then that I received a phone call from Doris who resided in independent living, warden controlled care facility and rang requiring emotional support. Doris would ring the Nursing together every day just for the company. "Hello Chris Nurse together," "Oh hi Chris it's nice to hear your voice, you must be new. I want to talk to you about my friend Samantha she said she can't wait for me to hit the bucket and go to my funeral! What do you suggest? She asked.

"I would advise you to try to ignore her as she does not seem very kind," I advised. "It's a bit lonely here, when the carers are gone I have no one to speak to, I spend most of my time looking out of the window, watching the mother next door playing with her infant children, I wish I wasn't so alone," she sighed.

"Can you not ring your sister, I can see from our previous notes that you listed her as next of kin?" I enquired trying to resolve her loneliness.
"Oh Chris I'm watching my favorite film she's just jumped back on the boat the silly cow, oh she is daft, have you seen it, it's about that boat that sunk years ago it's called shipwrecked," she began. "Oh you mean Titanic I like that film."

I felt so disheartened listening to Doris on the phone, so many elderly people in the UK are on their own. During a typical day, she would meet her carers, and speak to her sister on the phone, but she felt isolated. She stared out of the window remember her past with a deep sense of loneliness, missing her daughter who passed away. Ringing nurse together enabled Doris to build that emotional connection she was longing for.

In the afternoon I went in the car with nurse Maria to visit the clients we had contacted in the morning who required urgent care, or needed a nursing assessment to help prevent hospital admission. I stepped into Maria's orange car and witnessed her terrible driving. Maria constantly swore throughout the car journey whilst playing Cliff Richard's greatest hits.

We visited the first house of Deborah, the elderly lady who had dementia and was unable to remember her family contact details, who I believed had a fall during the phone call. We arrived at her address at
1 pm a small rural cottage in Yorkshire. The carers let us in the house, and I was shocked as I walked in. Deborah was sitting in her rocking chair with her feet on a footrest watching daytime tv. "Hello Deborah I'm Chris I rang you earlier, Did you have a fall earlier did you get help to go onto the toilet?" I asked. "Well I was shouting for my carer to come but she didn't answer, I got a bit muddled, I'm sorry to disturb you!" she smiled.
"Usually we write down a timetable for Deborah Of when we will visit her, but she lost it this morning and rang you for assistance, she tried to get up and fell on the wooden floor, so we bandaged her knee," smiled the young carer. I watched as Deborah looked so content in her rocking chair, I feared she had been injured. The carer arrived before the ambulance team assisted her.

We then made our way to the next patient's house, Donald Cranmore who lived with his wife Stella, the physiotherapist in our team John was already with him in the garden. "Oh quick please help us Donald went up on the ladders trying to put the bird's house on the top of the shed and fell." When we walked into the garden we found John laying on the patio floor, in his blue dungarees with his straw hat, he started to whine in pain, as we observed blood seeping through his trousers. "Oh bugger Stella why did you invite the cast of casualty into our house!" he shouted. "It's to help you Donald your always falling and you really need help!" Stella cried.

It was then that Mary rudely brushed past me with her light blue nursing bag, "Don't worry Donald I have a dressing that will heal your wound in no time." she smiled. I watched as Mary wobbled over to Donald, completing the non-touch technique, explaining to all of us how wonderful she was in completing it!

Once Donald's leg was dressed the physiotherapist John grabbed his MEGA bed device, a special blanket that is rolled underneath a patient and inflates to become a wheeled mattress in emergencies. We wheeled john into the house, whilst helping him to transfer to the bed with the aid of his three-wheeled walkers. As we arrived back in the house, we agreed with John and Stella that he would have carers come into the house, to help him with washing and dressing, and to continue to receive support from the physio rehab team on a weekly basis.

We then made our way to the final house for that afternoon, we visited Eileen who was struggling to look after her husband, Thomas, who was living with dementia. We arrived at her three-story mansion in a rural part of Yorkshire. Eileen stood at the entrance looking worried, she stood in her red gown, her grey curly hair towered above her hair, her face was pale, and she wore green glasses.

"Oh goodness thank God you came Thomas is outside now, he's smashing the greenhouse, you have to stop him!" she shouted. Mary comforted a shaken Eileen. As I walked through the house I looked on in shock, as smashed photographs were spread all over the living room floor. In the kitchen, broken plates and glass covered the entire floor.

I walked outside to find Thomas smashing the greenhouse with great anger. He stood with his spade wearing his blue pajamas, his green eyes were filled with anger. "Who are you? What are you doing in my house!" he shouted. "I am Chris a nurse I have come to help you," I offer. Suddenly Thomas flew into a fit of rage and aimed his spade towards me, "You lying bastard, you've come to rob me blind you skinny bastard!" he shouted. Thomas waved the spade in the air, but I managed to crawl to my feet, and ran towards the kitchen door. We had to barricade the kitchen door with the steel chairs as we called the emergency services. That afternoon Thomas was sectioned and taken to the local hospital, whilst we offered Eileen counseling support.

I found my first day emotionally draining, answering emotive calls, and dealing with distressing events in the community, without the aid of specialized equipment that a ward can offer.
I went home that afternoon and my parents had prepared a wonderful roast dinner, with a delicious chocolate cake cooking in the oven. It was then that I explained to my parents about Michael's son, Mum and Dad both cried at the news. Mum explained that she needed to go for a walk in the countryside, trying to absorb the shock of what she had heard. My parents had struggled to come to terms with Michael's death, spending their time traveling from country to country as a way of coping with their grief.

As I went upstairs I continued to place my brother's items into boxes, ready to put into the loft. I found so many items that gave a snapshot into his lonely life as a junior doctor, tickets to concerts he would book in the evenings, diary entries which included his frustrations at not passing his medical tests first time, details of letters which showed he had been attending counseling sessions for the depression he was seeking, believing he felt he was being forced into becoming a doctor.
I decided not to tell my parents about what I found, it was my brother's private messages, and I wanted them to preserve the good memories they had.

I arrived at the nurse together office ready to start my second day. I finally overcame my nerves and was ready to face the challenges. The office environment was calm and relaxing in comparison to the stressful ward environment. Each staff member in the office sat with a warm drink before they started work, and would talk about their weekend. It was so hard on the ward to ever enjoy a warm drink, conversations were usually rushed and focused on overcoming issues such as the shortage of staff on the wards, and the poor morale which affected the working environment.

I connected my phone and immediately it started to ring. "Hi, Nurse together how can I help you? Chris speaking."
"Oh hello Chris it's Doris, I'm glad it's you!" Doris beamed. Doris rang nurse together several times the previous day looking for emotional support, often becoming angry if a nurse attempted to end a call.
"Oh Chris I just had a carer come to this fat cow Lucy, oh dear she's a right mare telling me to eat my breakfast, so I told her to go on a diet! Here Chris what did you have for your breakfast?" she asked.
"Cornflakes," I responded. "How can I help you, Doris? Is there any way I can improve things for you?" I asked.

"No I'm done for now too old, I can't walk without my walker, I have no one to speak to," "you can always phone us, Doris you are never alone," I added. "Can we play a game? How about name this tune, hold on I'll get the radio," Doris beamed. I listened as Doris walked into the kitchen to get the radio, and she began to yawn on the phone. "Oh Doris you sound tired, do you want to have a rest first," I offered, then Doris abruptly hang up. It was so difficult as we tried desperately to help Doris but each initiative such as going to a community center she would refuse.

The phone started to ring, and I could hear instantly that the caller was upset. "Hi it's Deborah I'm ringing about my Mum Susan, she's a Type 2 Diabetic, she was discharged from hospital over two months ago, but her home situation is shocking. Mum has refused me to access her home for over a month. Mum's living room is cluttered in cat mess, with clothes and food spewed everywhere, she refuses for me to help clean her house, and I just found out she's sent a letter to the district nurse saying that she has moved, she's missed her medication, I've just rang and she admitted she needs help," Deborah cried, sobbing into the phone.

"Deborah, we can visit your mum later this afternoon as an urgent appointment to assess her, would that be ok?" I asked. "Yes thank you this is really going to make a difference!" she cheered.

It was a situation I had come across frequently in the past when I worked in the community patients, who lived in inhabitable conditions and refused to accept help, this was often due to depression, or the patient's inability to cope with their illnesses.

I observed the other three nurses I worked within the office that morning, Louisa Maria and Jenny. They were all so different and brought different strengths to the team. Louisa was upbeat and positive, but spent most of her time singing, running away from the phone calls to make a cup of tea. Jenny was constantly stressed, asking the other callers to be quiet if they were disturbing her whilst she was working, and would often bang her folders against the desk during a difficult call. Whilst Maria tented to raise her voice making sure everyone could hear and liked to retain a presence. Whilst I felt more relaxed in the office, the same pressures I felt in the ward existed, as I still had to meet work targets.

The phone continued to ring, a woman called Lisa rang who I had previously looked after on the stroke ward, who suffered an ischemic stroke, rang for support. "Hi, Chris I recognize your voice! How are you?" Lisa asked."
"I am very well Lisa how are you coping with life back at work after the stroke?" I asked.
I remembered Lisa worked as an Art lecturer in London, and her biggest fear after the stroke was her concern that she may not be able to draw again. After three months of intensive physiotherapy and occupational therapy, Lisa was able to walk again.

"Physically Chris I'm doing well but I am having serious difficulties with my memory. I am forgetting work appointments, the other morning I got lost going to work, and the most terrifying episode occurred on Saturday, I forgot where I parked my car whilst out shopping and it took me five hours to find it, the trouble is my car was at home! I forget that I had walked to the shops."

"Try not to worry Lisa memory problems can be directly caused by the stroke, would you like us to come out to see you this afternoon to try to help you?"

"Yes! Thank you, Chris, that would be so helpful.

As soon as I put the phone down the phone started to ring, "Hi it's Imelda here I need some support for my husband can you please help me, he is at the end stage of his lung cancer condition and he is in increased pain."

"Do you mind if we come to your house this afternoon to review the pain medication?"

"Yes Chris of course, but I feel like I can't cope I've got no support! Please help me!" she cried.

"Imelda please try to be strong, we will be at your home later offering support to both you and John" I cheered.

"I need to support my daughters have gone on holiday, and I'm by myself completing all the daily care tasks, I will be so grateful to see you," Imelda added.

As soon as the phone call ended, Jenny stood in the center of the room, her face was red with anger, and she looked fit to burst, she held onto her head in frustration. "Please can everyone please keep the volume down in this room, all I can hear loud unnecessary needs, this is not a playground!" she roared before storming out of the office to have her cigarette, as she swooped away in her black dress like a wicked witch. I was worried, as I was ordered to spend the afternoon attending home visits with Jenny, and she was already in a foul mood.

On my break I began to look for auditions online, in a few short months' time my time as a newly qualified nurse would come to an end, and I would have to choose my next path.

The phone started to ring, "Nurse together Chris How can I help you?" I asked.

"Hello Chris I am Amanda, I am ringing regarding my father Greg who has been diagnosed with Alzheimer's disease. My father is struggling to eat, he is up at night wandering keeping my mother awake, and he only responds to music. I feel he needs admiral nurse input.

"Tell me more about how music helps you father?"

"My Dad used to be a professional pianist and dancer, for over twenty years, he has not played. Now he sits at the piano playing all the music he learned when he left school including Beethoven and Mozart. My father played in symposiums and concert halls. Also as soon as we play music, he starts to dance and waltz with us in the room, but when he sits down he refuses to talk."

"Well, Amanda we can visit your house this afternoon to try to offer you father support with eating and drinking, and have a friend from our befriending company come to sit with your Dad to offer support.

It occurred to me whilst Amanda was on the phone the power that music had for people with dementia. When I looked after patients with dementia, putting on the radio to play a familiar song, would instantly help to alleviate their mood. Music was especially powerful for people with dementia as it helped patients to reminisce about moments in their lives and took them back to a happier time. Since my brother passed away I always struggled to listen to music that we listened to together including Oasis and the Beatles.

The phone started to ring and I could instantly hear a younger woman crying down the phone, "Please help me, I need some help desperately," she cried hysterically. "I am here to help you tell me your concerns," I offered. "It's my husband Joel yesterday he was bitten whilst we were sitting in the garden, today his leg is swollen, and he has a rash all over his body."

"Have you considered ringing the emergency services?" I asked. "No I can't ring the ambulance, he has a fear of hospitals, can you come round to see him try and treat him?" she asked. "Ok Jill we will put Joel on our urgent list for an afternoon visit today," I added. It was a difficult phone call as I had urged them to seek emergency help as they described the symptoms.

We then proceeded to visit Greg's house the man who was living with dementia but was struggling with eating and drinking, and his behavior had rapidly declined. Greg lived in a beautiful Edwardian three-story mansion. In the dining room, the white piano lay underneath the chandelier. As we walked in Greg proceeded to attack Jenny, as she was wearing a black coat he believed she was a parking attendant. "Oh fiddlesticks," she screamed, before we distracted Greg, by ushering him to the piano. As he started to play edelweiss on the piano he began to smile. Greg refused to answer any questions and appeared depressed when we initiated a conversation. When he played the piano his mood completely transformed. Amanda expressed further concerns about her father.

"I'm not sure we can have him live in our house for much longer, he has become more aggressive, attacking the postman with a baseball bat this morning, he also smashed the window of the shed with a spade as he saw his reflection in the glass window, and this evening he smashed the television on the floor, believing he could hear mysterious noises.

We explained that we could offer a social worker to discuss an assessment and a referral to a dietician to help with his meals. It was so sad to see how difficult life can be for families caring for their loved ones with dementia. Many of the patients in the community were unaware of support in the community such as carer support, activity groups, and admiral nurse input.

That afternoon I went to Jenny's car to start the afternoon shift with her. "Oh Chris you will need these to cover your shoes," she scowled, passing me a plastic bag to cover my shoes. The journey with Jenny that afternoon with Jenny was terrifying, she beeped the horn constantly. I felt terrified and uncomfortable throughout the journey, Jenny was so cantankerous and angry if I were to say the wrong word she would fly into a fit of rage.

We arrived at our first patient's house, Susan, the lady who had neglected herself in her own home. When we arrived it started to rain, Susan's daughter Deborah was waiting outside in the pouring rain, wearing her red anokorok, her blonde hair was soaked. Susan handed us the key and we made our way into the house. When we walked into the house the stench was unbearable, it smelt like strong horse manure. In the hallway hundreds of unopened letters. Then we entered the living room and I gasped in. Susan sat in the middle of the room in her red rocking chair, she was an obese lady with curlers in hair, blue glasses, and wore a beanie hat, and had a cigarette in her mouth. Susan was surrounded by piles of junk food, opened crisp packets, half-eaten burgers, green papers, hundreds of books and newspapers were scattered all over the floor. In the corner of the room was a little black and white kitchen.

In Susan's kitchen were over a dozen cats crawling in and out of the cupboards. I trudged through the piles of mess and knelt down to observe Susan's legs, covered in blisters that had almost turned necrotic. Susan began to cry as she held onto my hand, "I'm so sorry I'm so embarrassed, of you both seeing this, I know I need help, I'm just so scared!" She sobbed.

"Susan you've made the right step, you've called us it's the first step in getting you practical help." As I knelt before her Jenny handed me the dressing pack and I put a dressing on her ulcerative legs.

"My life changed after my husband was killed in a car accident two years ago, and I've given up, I've let depression take over me, I've pushed you away to Deborah," she sobbed into her handkerchief. I then held onto Susan's hand to let her know I was there for her and in that instant that this was the true essence of nursing, supporting people in their darkest moments, and letting people know you are always here for them.

When I took Susan's blood sugar reading was abnormally low, and her ECG presented to us that she had an abnormal heart rhythm. Susan agreed that afternoon to go to A and E to take the first step in getting the care she desperately needed.

We then proceeded to go to Lisa's house, the former stroke patient I cared for as a student nurse. When We entered Lisa's luxury two-bedroom studio apartment I looked on in awe. The apartment was filled with wonderful paintings she had drawn, including a detailed intricate drawing, of a wedding couple walking into the sunset, whilst another drawing was of the twin towers.

It was amazing to see how talented she was. On the ward stroke patient, Lisa had lost all movement in her hands and struggled to physically hold her pencil. Lisa sat at the dining table explaining her memory difficulties, including getting lost on her way home from her run.

I then completed a mini mental health test which is a cognition test, which is written to test for conditions such as dementia. The test involved arithmetic, remembering words, and answering questions related to date and time. Lisa had passed the initial test but explained that she had felt a tingling sensation she experienced two years ago before she had a stroke. We booked Lisa to have an urgent brain scan the next day and for a consultation with the stroke consultant.

The third house we visited was Imelda and John's house. John was in the late stages of his cancer illness. We walked into their spacious bungalow, everything was white including the carpet and walls. John lay in his double bed in the dining room facing the patio window to the entrance of the garden. John lay in his blue pajamas, his face was so angelic in appearance, He was so polite and content despite his prognosis. On the walls were photos that showed the journey of his life. Including a picture of John as a seventeen-year-old soldier. Whilst the other picture showed him with his wife on his wedding day, and another photo showed john wearing meeting the Queen to receive his knighthood.

I sat on the bed next to John, "How can we help make things better for you at home? Is there any way we can help you?" I asked.
"Well I would like my pain medication reviewed, and I want to have oxygen at home as I'm finding that I'm struggling to breathe and it becomes worse on exertion. I would also need a carer to help me in the morning as my wife is struggling to get me dressed in the morning."

"Well we can help you we can discuss your care needs with the social worker, and look into prescribing oxygen at home to help improve your breathing," I began.
It was an honor spending the time with John, talking about ways to improve his quality of life, and talking about his army days, leaving his home and girlfriend at quality of seventeen, and finally returning home at twenty one and commencing his training as a doctor. As John lay in bed he had a beautiful view of

the garden, with a six-foot water fountain, and garden. John had come to terms with his prognosis and was appreciative of our help.

My time in the community was both an exciting and hectic experience. I learned so much about the lives of our patients when they return home. Working as a community nurse offers a unique insight into the personal lives of the patients. I enjoyed the relaxed nature of working in the office and being able to take my breaks uninterrupted. Speaking on the phone to people was a huge barrier, and I always felt like I was not given the full picture of the patient's situation.

CHAPTER 9: MY BROTHER'S SECRET DIARY

Before I started my final rotation I was given two weeks' annual leave. I always found time away from work difficult, I would spend most of my time trying to distract myself from thoughts about my brother Micheal. Every part of the house would remind me of him, his room which was left untouched, our garden where we would play football, and various photos of me and Micheal were present in each room of the house. To unwind and take my mind off the grieving process, I would ride my bike through the Yorkshire country fields, watch a movie in town, and when I arrived home I would write stories in the study.

On this day I could not seem to focus and sat in the dining room watching home videos of holidays and special events I shared with my brother. I watched the video of Micheal and me singing our favorite Oasis and Keane songs in his private hospital room, following his chemotherapy treatment. I then watched the trip we undertook traveling across the USA, including New York, Florida, and the Grand Canyon.

I watched the scene, in which we stood over the cliff top of a mountain in the Grand Canyon. I remember that moment standing on the clifftop with Micheal, the view was breathtaking, all we could hear was the whistling of the wind. From the cliff edge we could view the mountains in the distance, glistening as the sun began to set, the only company we had were the white doves swooping above us. At that moment on top of the cliff, we promised each other that we would come back to America on our 28th Birthday, as part of our trip around the world. I never planned or imagined my life without Micheal, now that he was gone, I felt like all of my dreams and plans were frozen, I was lost in time.

That afternoon I went into my brother's room and picked up his diary that he had written during his years as a junior doctor, I felt compelled to read it, and spent the day sitting at his desk learning all about the life he had kept hidden. In the first entries of the diary, he detailed his difficult transition to Belfast to start his training as a junior doctor. Many of the medical students would go into the O' leary pub at night next to the Belfast college. Micheal would spend his evenings studying, researching different conditions, he had been taking medication recklessly to cope with his crippling anxiety dew pressure he felt.

Micheal detailed that he was so nervous for the objective structured clinical examinations that he couldn't sleep or eat, and felt disheartened when he had to resist a practical examination.

Micheal's experiences on the medical and surgical wards parallelled the experiences I had been through as a student nurse. During his first rotation on a general medical ward, he detailed that the consultant would constantly ask him questions on the spot, and throw folders on the ground if he was to answer a question wrong. A register who worked alongside Micheal had attempted to get him thrown off the ward, simply because he did not like working in close proximity with junior doctors. I had been through the same as a student nurse, working alongside mentors who were too busy to offer guidance to support me, and even worked with a nurse who despised students and made my life hell.

However, despite Micheal's difficulty under the bureaucracy, he faced in his close-knit team, he achieved great strides as a doctor. In his diary Micheal listed his achievements in the ward, such as saving the life of a girl with epilepsy, helping to deliver a baby of a woman who had barricaded herself in the hospital toilets. Micheal had also participated in emergency CPR and had to break the bad news to his patients which he felt heightened his anxiety.

Micheal also spoke of his minor failures as a student, such as accidentally leaving a catheter bag lead open, causing urine to spill on the floor, and his senior consultant to fall onto the floor. Micheal also struggled when he failed his first clinical observation.

In Micheal's dairy, he detailed his particular interest in working with patients who had dementia. Our Grandfather James was an accountant and developed Alzheimer's disease at the age of eighty. We watched our Grandfathers personality change from a happy, vibrant, hardworking man, to a quiet angry suspicious person. The hardest part of our Grandfather suffering from Alzheimer's disease was watching him losing his independence. In his final days, James lay in his bed in the guest room overlooking Boulmer beach.

Micheal detailed in his diary that he had continued to complete research-based around dementia, and he intended to be part of the fix dementia campaign and had a dream of working with other doctors to find a cure or a definite preventative measure.

What I found most difficult about reading Micheal's diary was the loneliness he felt going to the cinema his own, and feeling that his medication for depression had inhibited his feelings to want to make friends. It was not until Micheal met Susan that he found true happiness, and they would spend time together, going to the beach, riding their bikes down country roads, and singing together in bars.

As I read through Micheal's diary that day it made me grateful that he had lived a very full life. I felt like I was uncovering his private life. I was not aware at the time that Micheal had intended for his friends and family to know more about his life as a doctor.

CHAPTER 10:
CHRISTMAS EVE
IN A AND E

I was terrified when my final rotation ward was announced on an Accident and Emergency ward at the Yorkshire hospital. I had always feared I wouldn't be able to cope with the fast-paced nature of working in A and E, as I enjoyed the structure of planned admissions on the ward I worked on.

My first day on the accident and Emergency ward was on Christmas Eve. The A and E department consisted of a circular shape. The nurse's station was in the middle of the bay with the sixteen nursing cubicles formed a circle around the station.

As I walked onto the ward I witnessed the hysteria and buzz of energy. Three Patients lying on trolleys were waiting by the station with the paramedics to be admitted. The nursing station was filled with doctors making notes and nurses making phone calls. The nurses on the ward were rushing around, completing a variety of tasks such as blood tests, ECGs and patient observations. Patients were shouting out for help, buzzes were ringing constantly, it was like disorganized chaos, and I felt so lost!

I finally met my supervisor Abby a thirty-year-old newly qualified nurse, she was six foot four with mousy brown curly hair and wore green glasses. "Hi Chris pleasure to meet you, if you take cubicles one to five for today I would be grateful, you need to do full admission, blood, ECG, etc." She explained, before disappearing behind a curtain. I had so many questions to ask her on my first day, where do I find all the equipment I need? Abby was so busy, so stressed, she didn't have the time to help.

The first patient was Shelly a seventy-three-year-old lady admitted by her sister with confusion, Shelley sat in the hospital chair wearing her pink dirty dressing gown with holes in her slippers, her skin was tanned and her hair seemed to tower over her head, greasy with a smell of cigarettes. Shelley sat looking vacantly into the distance. Shelly's sister Karen stood in a green suit next to her.

"Oh nurse She really needs help, I've been to America for three months since I returned her behavior has completely changed. I'm hearing from the neighbors that she is up till 3 am at night singing in her garden, she is struggling with her driving and crashed into the back of a post van, her neighbor witnessed her shaving her cat when she visited her house. Ever since her husband died six months ago she hasn't spoken," Karen sighed. I then walked over to Shelley to take her blood pressure, "Can I take your blood pressure?" I asked. "Go away from me little boy, Go away!" she squealed, kicking the trolley out of the way.

"Shelley, you need to calm down you're disturbing the other patients" Karen warned. Shelley then proceeded to stand up and knocked the cups from the drink trolley angrily on the floor, before mistaking a woman's bag for her own. Shelley snatched the bay from a very uptight middle-aged woman who was in the cubicle with her pregnant daughter. "That's my bag!" shouted the lady. "No it's mine you thieving bitch!" she shouted running around the ward. "Shelley can you sit down for a second so we can have a talk," I pestered. I walked after Shelley who was nervously looking for the front door, whilst the angry middle-aged woman followed her.

When Shelley attempted to escape the security guard furiously ushered her back into the ward. After much persuasion, Shelley returned the bag to the middle-aged woman. I arranged for the healthcare assistant to supervise Shelley on a one to one basis, whilst she was waiting to be transferred to the hospital mental health ward for assessment.

I then turned to my patient in cubicle two a forty-two-year-old man named Chris, who at thirty stone was clinically obese, and was admitted following a heart attack. Chris sat holding the hand of his elderly mother Dora, who looking terrified, shaking in her grey mint coat, as he began to cry with his oxygen mask on. "Chris was so successful two years ago, flying around the world as an executive accountant, then after his wife Laura passed, he fell into a deep depression, and spent most of his time eating junk food and drinking heavily. "I completed clinical observations on Chris and discovered that his heart rate and breathing rate was causing clinical concern. I looked at Chris as tears rolled down his pale face, as he held onto my hand. "I don't want any treatment please, I've just given up, my wife passed away and I can't cope on my own, let me die!" he pleaded. Suddenly the sister on the ward

Katy Ann arranged for the porters to take Chris to the intensive care ward for closer observation.

Life as a nurse in the accident and emergency ward appeared very stressful. There was no structure on the ward, and as looked around all I could see was chaos. Ten beds were lined up outside of the A and E department, an elderly man was banging his walking stick along the nurse's desk to get his attention, and nurses and health care assistants seemed to run around in anger.

After my lunch break, a middle-aged man walked in wearing his suit, his face was red, his lips were swollen, he appeared confused and disoriented. I held the man by the hand and ushered him to sit on the green recliner chair. "Hello I'm Chris I will be looking after you," I explained. He began to appear more disorientated and his speech became slurred. "I've been stung," he muttered, as his breathing became slower and labored. I realized instantly that the man was suffering from an anaphylaxis reaction, and I helped to sit him up to help control the pattern of his breathing.
I then nervously ran for the anaphylaxis treatment book which contained an injection with epinephrine (adrenaline) to help relieve his allergic response. I administered the injection, whilst Andy started to shiver and sweat profusely. I Put an oxygen mask to give him oxygen, and Abby appeared and helped to set up intravenous fluids which contained antihistamines to help improve his breathing.

As soon as I administered the injection and antihistamine Bill's breathing rate returned to normal, the redness in his face gradually reduced, and the swelling in his lip reduced rapidly. It was then that Bill grabbed onto my hand, "thank you, Chris, for all of your support, you've saved my life!" he beamed. I then organized for Bill to stay in the acute medical ward for further observation until the symptoms were more controlled and he was fit to go home.

It did not feel like Christmas Eve at all, I was nervous, scared, and anxious in the Accident and Emergency department and felt like I was being thrown into the deep end. Abby was busy completing her own tasks, and every time I would try to engage in conversation with the senior sisters, they were called away to assess a patient or to check the bed state.

I thought about the previous Christmas Eve performing in Broadway in California in front of five thousand people. I was so happy, so relaxed, surrounded by my friends and work-family. I had nearly come to the end of my newly qualified year and I felt like I was lost under a sea of paperwork and ward drama.

At 5 pm a young boy aged seventeen came in after participating in a football match, he walked in holding his chest, wearing blue dungarees, his wild brown curly hair flopped over his head, wearing his bright blue glasses. I could see him start to wince in pain, I walked him over to the blue chair in cubicle 3. "Hello I'm Chris I'm the nurse who will be looking after you, can I take your name?" I asked.

"I'm Sean I was just playing football in the park across the road and I started to have chest pains, I'm worried as my father passed away when I was little from a heart attack," he murmured. "Please try not to worry Sean I will help you," I promised. As he lay on the bed I completed blood and conducted a blood test and completed an ECG. Sean looked at me with tears in his eyes as he began to cry, passing his phone to me, "can you tell my mum that I'm here she will be worried sick," he cried. As I rang the mum I could hear the fear in her voice as she explained she was on her way. The ECG showed that Sean had an abnormal heart rhythm. "Am I going to be Ok Chris You will help me?" he asked looking at me helplessly. I turned around to grab the attention of the doctor when suddenly, Chris fell off the bed and collapsed onto the floor in agony. "Help!" I shouted. Sean was now unconscious on the cold hospital floor. Suddenly I was surrounded by a sea of doctors, nurses, and two student nurses. I checked Sean's airway and attempted to rouse him by verbally talking to him.

It was then that I started to complete the thirty compressions, I was sweating and shaking. I have to save him, I have to say this young teenager, I can't allow him to die I thought. I was completely surrounded by a range of medical professionals, as Abby brought the Crash trolley to the scene, taking over the compressions, desperately trying to save his life. I looked on in fear wondering how I would explain this to Sean's mother.

Suddenly Sean's Mum appeared on the ward, trying to make her way through the crowds, dressed as an Elf coming from her works Christmas party. She made her way nervously to the front panicking, instantly collapsing onto the ground in front of her son, whilst nurse Abby tried to hold her back. The resister and resuscitation team tried desperately to revive him, but sadly their efforts didn't work, Sean died at 6 pm that evening. Sean had died from an undiagnosed heart murmur, and I felt so devastated, knowing that he had all his life in front of him, later discovering that he was signed to a professional football club.

That afternoon Sean's mother Patricia sat in the nurse's office, crying, explaining she wanted to speak to me, she held onto my held trembling. "I want to thank you for being with my son in his final hours, I am so grateful he was with such a kind and caring nurse, this is not your fault," she cried, holding me tight. A tear rolled down my cheek, this was the true essence of being a nurse, supporting people through the darkest of times offering support and empathy.

The three months I spent in on the Accident and Emergency were the most difficult times I had spent as a nurse. I had completed CPR on several patients, helped to support staff when several patients were brought in, following a major road traffic incident and broken up a fight between two men on the ward who attempted to kill each other with weapons. I found it incredibly difficult to think quickly, to problem solve, I felt much more comfortable in the ward, being able to plan nursing care.

CHAPTER 11: THE FINAL GOODBYE

I could finally relax after a stressful year I had finally completed my year as a newly qualified nurse, and was now looking forward to the future.

My 28th birthday arrived, and it was a pivotal day that changed my life forever.

I woke up on a bright Sunday morning, the sun cast a shadow over my face, as the winter cold made me shiver. I walked downstairs and when I walked into the dining room I observed a dozen presents on the oak table. The gifts included a robot, a photo album of unseen photos from past family holidays, and holiday vouchers. My parents and I both found it so difficult to celebrate my birthday in my brother's absence, but it was a way of celebrating his memory.]

I became quite suspicious on my birthday as my parents had explained they were going to travel to London to visit my nephew, but they explained that I needed to open up the mysterious envelope Micheal had left me at 3 pm. I wondered if they knew what the contents were.

At 2 pm I entered the Kitchen and mum had decorated the table with a happy birthday tablecloth and filled the table with beautiful turkey, roast potatoes, and a glistening chocolate gateau. My mother had just gone upstairs. I went over to the sink to make myself a glass of water when I turned around the turkey was gone! I looked out of the kitchen window and found out chocolate labrador dog Polly galloping down the harden with the turkey. By the time I reached her, she had devoured the entire turkey and let out an enormous burp. My birthday meal was ruined, my parents were furious for my carelessness in letting Polly in. That afternoon we sat around the hot warm fire and had chicken noodle soup before my parents left for their journey to visit my nephew.

It was finally time for me to open up my brother's red envelope. I started to tremble and could feel my heart racing with fear. Inside the envelope were a DVD, a cheque for five thousand pounds, a list of tasks to complete, and a mysterious script called 'the doctor. '

I put the DVD on and looked on in wonder as I watched my brother sitting on the edge of his hospital bed explaining his wishes for me. He was wearing his white hospital gown, attached to a drip, having just undergone a grueling chemotherapy session. "If you're watching this video like I requested, it will be our 28th birthday, the second birthday you've celebrated after my passing. I made this video to explain my final hopes and wishes for you. I've arranged for Tom and Tim to come to your house tonight for a reunion, it will be good for you to see them. You do not have to be alone. Inside the envelope I have a bucket list for you to complete ten things before you're 30, I want you to take on challenges and push yourself! Finally, find my script 'the doctor' it's my journey through medical school, and I was hoping maybe one day you can turn it into a play! Anyway, Chris, it's goodbye from me I hope you have a wonderful life!" he beamed before the screen faded to black.

It finally felt that I could begin the process of moving on with my life, the DVD message gave me the push I needed to realize I had to move on. Micheal left a list of tasks for me to complete such as, complete a Bungee jump, make friends with two strangers, write a book, and complete the London marathon. I was so happy to have his script 'the doctor' it felt like I had a piece of Micheal with me forever. My old childhood friends Tim and Tom arrived that afternoon and we went bowling.

Two weeks later I had attended an audition to play Captain Von Trapp in the Sound of Music production at Broadway. I successfully won the part.
I was back in my role as an actor and for the first time in my life, I was happy for the future.
Nursing was one of the most exciting and challenging journeys of my life. I faced many challenges working on the wards as a nurse. I was delegating to other staff, I supervised students, I practically ran wards when they were short-staffed, and I watched people recover and held their hands in their final moments. It was a privilege to look after the sick and to make a difference in people's lives. Once you become a nurse you see the world differently, and I truly believe if you constantly hold the values of honesty,

compassion, kindness and empathy and never lose hold of these values, you will continue to make a difference.

CHAPTER 12: TIPS FOR A NEWLY QUALIFIED NURSE

Remember to still ask questions learning is continuous throughout your nursing journey.

Always make sure to take regular breaks, skipping breaks will cause fatigue and affect your performance.

If you feel you are not enjoying your first nursing post, remember that there are many opportunities to work in other areas, once you spend a year in your post begin looking for other posts suited to you.

If your trust runs a weekly nurse forum, make sure you attend it can be a great experience to meet newly qualified and experienced nurses, share your experiences and learn from them.

Make sure you get six to eight hours of sleep each night, this will help to prevent burnout.

Be open and honest in staff meetings, if you feel something needs to change in the ward, report it, and you could be making a difference.

Make sure you take time out for yourself after a shift, go for a walk, listening to music and going to the gym, it is important to have time out.

Do not get into a pattern of working late every shift, working late can often go unnoticed and only causes stress.

In your appraisal meetings make sure you are aware of any further training opportunities open to you and take part in this.

Delegate carefully and fairly make sure each staff member is competent to complete a task given to them if they make a mistake it could affect your career.

Always report bullying, ignoring bullying in a hospital work setting can lead to depression and anxiety. Speak to your manager about any concerns, to avoid escalation of the bullying.

Make sure you are signed up to a union.

Do not accept violence if you feel physically threatened on the ward call security.

If you are involved in a CPR incident, try to seek feedback from the hospital resuscitation team. It is always helpful to know how you can improve your skills.

Always try to smile and remain positive to your patients, I have worked with nurses who appear hostile due to home circumstances, make sure home and work lives are kept very separate.

Always report poor practice as soon as you see it, if you see tablets left unattended, or a staff member not completing the correct manual handling procedure, make sure you speak up.

Try and eat a healthy and balanced diet, eating unhealthy foods can be tempting when working unsociable hours.

If you feel you are struggling or not receiving the right support in your newly qualified year, tell your manager immediately.

When you are giving medications try to avoid distractions, if a staff member needs help, delegate the task to another staff member, distractions can lead to medication errors

As a newly qualified nurse try and keep a journal of your shifts, it can be therapeutic to write about your experiences and to learn from them.

In your appraisal ask for constructive feedback.

Visit other nursing areas in your newly qualified year it can help to broaden your knowledge and help you decide if you want to work in another area.

If you feel stressed or at risk of burnout seek help immediately from your GP support is available to help you.

Thank you for reading my book if you enjoyed it leave a review!

Connect with me on instagram @buttinchris
Connect with me on twitter: @christo25288316

Printed in Great Britain
by Amazon